DEAR DR. SHAH!
THIS BOOK IS WRITTEN
FOR THOSE WHO CARE.
YOSEF D. D.
3/31/04

Dear S.
Thanks
making the way
in Quality
Andrea Pestito

Such a
pleasure to
know someone
who values what is
important for
making a difference
Sue Greenwood

The Quality Handbook for Health Care Organizations

Yosef D. Dlugacz

Andrea Restifo

Alice Greenwood

The Quality Handbook for Health Care Organizations

A Manager's Guide to
Tools and Programs

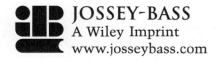

JOSSEY-BASS
A Wiley Imprint
www.josseybass.com

Published by Jossey-Bass
A Wiley Imprint
989 Market Street, San Francisco, CA 94103-1741   www.josseybass.com

Jossey-Bass books and products are available through most bookstores. To contact Jossey-Bass directly call our Customer Care Department within the U.S. at 800-956-7739, outside the U.S. at 317-572-3986, or fax 317-572-4002.

Jossey-Bass also publishes its books in a variety of electronic formats. Some content that appears in print may not be available in electronic books.

Library of Congress Cataloging-in-Publication Data

Dlugacz, Yosef D., 1947–
The quality handbook for health care organizations : a manager's guide to tools and programs / Yosef D. Dlugacz, Andrea Restifo, Alice Greenwood.— 1st ed.
p. ; cm.
Includes bibliographical references and index.
ISBN 0-7879-6921-4 (alk. paper)
1. Health services administration. 2. Health facilities—Personnel management. 3. Medical care—Quality control.
[DNLM: 1. Quality Assurance, Health Care—organization & administration—United States. 2. Critical Pathways—United States. 3. Data Collection—methods—United States. 4. Data Interpretation, Statistical—United States. 5. Quality Indicators, Health Care—United States. W 84 AA1 D626q 2004] I. Restifo, Andrea, 1965- II. Greenwood, Alice. III. Title.
RA971.35.D58 2004
362.1'1'0685—dc22
2003018922

Printed in the United States of America
FIRST EDITION
HB Printing   10 9 8 7 6 5 4 3 2 1

─᷍᷍᷍᷍᷍᷍᷍᷍— Contents

～～ Figures and Tables

Figures

Tables

─✺─ Foreword

In my experience during the past half century as chairman emeritus
of the Board of Governors and the Board of Regents, president and
president emeritus of the American College of Physicians, and serv-
ing on President Clinton's White House Review Group on health care
reform, I have seen firsthand the quantum change that has occurred
in how society receives and perceives health care, not only because of
new technologies but, what is more important, because of the pro-
gressive increase in medical knowledge and the application of scientific principles to medical care. Although the quest for excellence and
quality has been integral to this journey from the outset, it has benefited from the logical application of scientific, data-based information
to quality management initiatives. The *Quality Handbook for Health
Care Organizations* documents striking examples of this phenomenon
and provides an extraordinary road map to the pathways for improving health care services and responding to human health needs.

Literature is blessed with numerous publications describing quality programs in industry, the service sector, the military, and educational institutions, as well as in the health field. Although each is
important, none, other than caring for the health of our fellow humans, can be characterized as a calling. Health professionals have entered into a treasured covenant to serve those in need and to address
their welfare and well-being. There is little doubt that the weight of
this responsibility bears heavily on those entrusted with this charge,
who seek reliable, reproducible methods to ensure quality as an essential imperative for health care.

The scientific and data-based methodology of quality management
is discussed fully in this handbook; it employs knowledge, organization, and structure to achieve its objectives. This approach is rooted
in the history of the health professions, particularly in medicine, with
the early-twentieth-century work of Dr. Abraham Flexner, who in-
sisted on instilling the scientific method into the medical schools of

the United States, where little existed before. This history has repeated itself in the development of performance improvement activities and quality management initiatives. Central to this publication is the application of scientific discipline to the task at hand.

The reader of this handbook will discover some very special contributions to the field of quality management. Throughout its ten chapters, the authors take a hands-on approach to specific topics: the implementation of managerial leadership, the definition of accurate data, the clarification of required measurements, the exploration of new tools and techniques, and the complex integration of data into performance improvement objectives. Additionally, you will find numerous examples of clinical pathways and methods for ensuring appropriate hierarchical oversight of clinical and quality activities as well as logical solutions for addressing and preventing adverse events. Most important, the persuasive and beneficial principles of quality management in health care are firmly embedded in each chapter and expressed through clear, data-supported concepts.

In addition to the development of statistical methodology for retrospective and prospective review, a mainstay of performance improvement and the acceptance of regulatory oversight, there is, of course, the human element involved in delivering health care services. Throughout this handbook, the authors discuss human interactions, wrapped in trust, knowledge, and leadership. This is best expressed by the authors themselves: Yosef D. Dlugacz, Ph.D., Andrea Restifo, R.N., M.P.A., and Alice Greenwood, Ph.D., each an effective advocate of excellence in medical and nursing care and all good friends to quality performance. Dr. Dlugacz brings particular expertise to this enterprise through intelligence, tirelessness, persuasiveness, and vision. As senior vice president of quality management for the North Shore–Long Island Jewish Health System, he has demonstrated these attributes consistently to physicians, nurses, directors of quality management, pharmacists, administrators, and patients. He and his colleagues are indispensable agents in ensuring the quality of medical care, not only to those served by his health system but across the nation and abroad.

Although intended for middle and upper management personnel in health care facilities, this handbook should be attractive to all health professionals and is highly instructive for physicians and nurses in training and for medical and nursing students as well. The organization, descriptions, and content of the handbook reflect the types of analyses that one should consider as models in planning, implementing, and carrying out a multitude of performance improvement activities.

For more than a decade, I have observed firsthand the development of a sophisticated quality management program by these individuals across a large health system. The authors compare most favorably with their colleagues, regionally and nationally, and I am pleased to confirm their expertise in the field of quality management. The handbook is a well-constructed and well-defined reference; its teachings and methods will have a most positive effect on patients and those seeking health care. It is yet another support of the covenant to serve the health of the public and to meet the challenge of a calling for all its health professionals.

Lawrence Scherr, M.D., MACP
Betsey Cushing Whitney Dean and
Senior Vice President, Academic Affairs,
North Shore–Long Island Jewish Health System
Professor of Medicine,
New York University School of Medicine

This book is dedicated to all those who care.

~~~ Author's Note

This book is the product of twenty-five years' experience working in health care quality. Throughout this time I have been passionately committed to patient advocacy, to ensuring that every patient receives the very best services possible, delivered in an atmosphere of respect, dignity, and kindness. Reaching this goal has not been easy. It has been a long and arduous road to travel, refining my ideas and imposing them on many people along the way, but at the end I have seen the Quality Management Department transformed from a small office with the responsibility for maintaining compliance with regulatory requirements to the core and heartbeat of the organization, promoted and supported by its leadership and recognized as having a scientific methodology for evaluating processes and improving patient outcomes.

The institution has grown from a single hospital to one of the largest and most successful multihospital systems in the country today, in large part because of this commitment to and understanding of quality. Quality care involves more than tools, techniques, methods, and even outcomes. Quality requires a certain mindset, and not a complicated one at that: Do No Harm.

Of course I have not made this journey alone. The generosity of many physicians, nurses, managers of various departments, administrative leaders, and ancillary services staff in educating me about the delivery of care has helped me define and refine my ideas. I thank them all. As a sociologist, I was trained to extract underlying principles and to objectively evaluate alternative methods of providing health care services; this training has served me well. Integrating the information of so many dedicated health care providers into the quality management structure has benefited us all—the patients, the institution, and the caregivers—because working within a quality framework encourages doing the right thing.

Without the vision of two extraordinary CEOs, Michael J. Dowling and John S. T. Gallagher, and the commitment of the Board of Trustees to promote quality care, the Quality Management Department might still be merely translating regulatory requirements. Due to their insight and forward-looking perspective, delivering quality care has become a fundamental principle of the entire health care system.

Y.D.D.

~~ Preface

With the publication of the two Institute of Medicine books, *To Err Is Human* (1999) and *Crossing the Quality Chasm* (2001), the delivery of safe quality care has rocketed to the forefront of national attention. The health care services industry is being scrutinized, measured, evaluated, and publicized as never before, and an increasingly educated public expects to receive nothing less than excellent care and services. Gone are the days when a physician working in isolation dictated care to an unquestioning patient who had little choice about which hospital or health care facility to enter.

Today, health care professionals are accountable to the public they serve, with government and regulatory agencies monitoring every aspect of the delivery of care, as well as to the economic dictates of reimbursement policies. Government, regulatory agencies, and insurance payors expect health services to be rigorously measured within a quality framework and reported publicly. These "report cards" of hospital services and patient outcomes are splashed across the media, often with immediate economic consequences to those institutions whose reports reveal success or the lack of it in some aspect of the provision of care. Without undue exaggeration, it can be said that the twenty-first century is the dawn of a new era in health care, an era of accountability.

In this highly visible arena, managers and supervisors of health care services have more responsibility than ever before, both to their patients and to the organization that employs them. A great deal of pressure is associated with this responsibility, because poor management can lead to deficits in patient care and increased patient risk, and can even financially cripple an organization. Health care management is further complicated by the fact that most health care managers are promoted from within the ranks of the health care organization and have had little opportunity to be schooled in ways to function effectively and successfully to meet the requirements of today's health industry. Although some books target specific areas associated with the delivery of services, such as data analysis techniques, regulatory requirements, resource evaluation, fiscal management, and strategic planning, no book provides overarching theoretical and practical information to assist health care leaders, supervisors, managers, and staff with their daily responsibilities.

The *Quality Handbook for Health Care Organizations: A Manager's Guide to Tools and Programs* is designed to fill this gap, offering a practical and useful guide to quality management and providing information about the basic principles, methods, and the objective tools necessary for survival—and success—in today's complex health care industry. Quality management texts often focus on translating regulatory requirements into practical form or offer theoretical essays on the issues involved in the delivery of excellent patient care. But our daily experience in integrating quality and standardizing care across the eighteen-hospital North Shore–Long Island Jewish Health System (NS-LIJHS), one of the largest not-for-profit health care systems in the nation, has taught us that managers are eager to have actual models, methods, and tools to help them do their daily work.

Although the government, through its regulatory bodies, defines the function of the director, manager, supervisor, or leader and sets expectations for performance, it doesn't describe what the job entails or how to do it. Our experiences with direct patient care, with the analysis of adverse outcomes, and with regulatory agencies have illuminated the range of problems that managers have managing their services. The role of the manager is evolving; today's manager is not satisfied simply waiting for instructions and direction from above about how to do the job but takes a proactive approach to managing a unit or service and makes independent and informed decisions regarding the delivery of care.

The *Quality Handbook* will provide managers with the practical tools, techniques, and methods they need to make the best decisions for and deliver the best care to their patients. Our goal is to offer information that will assist them in carrying out their responsibilities. By learning how to collect and analyze quality information and data, and becoming familiar with the methods that are used to assess and implement change, managers and supervisors of various departments (Quality Management, Risk Management, Nursing, Nursing Education, Finance, Nutrition, Social Work, and Pharmacy, to name only a few) will learn to prioritize improvement efforts, evaluate resource consumption, produce intelligent reports for their departments and their own managers and supervisors, comply with regulatory requirements, conceptualize how their department interacts with the rest of the organization, and implement and sustain successful processes. Quality management techniques help health care providers and administrators to plan, direct, coordinate, provide, and improve health care services that respond to patient needs, promote desirable outcomes, and are cost-effective.

Furthermore, as health care institutions are charged by state and national regulatory agencies to do quality management in order to be accredited and receive Medicare reimbursement, individual departments have to have explicit processes and procedures in place to evaluate care and promote safe practices. Although they are required to work within a quality management framework, most health care workers have little access to information about what that means. The *Quality Handbook* will provide that information. The framework provided by the Joint Commission on Accreditation of Healthcare Organizations (JCAHO), the national accrediting agency for health care services, does more than require documentation of services. If interpreted appropriately, the regulations offer managers an outline for delivering excellent care and advocating for their patients.

It is impossible to deal with the vastness of the health care industry, with human resources, the environment of care, risk and legal issues, quality regulations, planning and finance, information systems, the medical boards, and so on, without a unifying theory and appropriate methods, tools, and models. Quality care, an abstract notion that most hospitals and networks articulate as part of their mission statements, needs to be made concrete and operationalized so that managers can incorporate the concept into the services they deliver. Quality management provides a theoretical model on which to base decisions, a rationale for prioritizing resources, a methodology for assessing and improving output, and a principled rhetoric that explains to managers or supervisors why they do what they do. This book will help health care managers make decisions that are consistent with their goals and capable of objective validation.

Learning to use quality information and data to promote services and having a framework to use that data to continually improve patient care are the tools managers need to do their jobs. This handbook outlines how to define, collect, aggregate, and analyze quality information to support intelligent decision making and deliver superior services. Those responsible for the delivery of care will be introduced to explicit performance improvement methodologies and to the tools that are useful for assessing and analyzing a variety of problems.

OUTLINE OF THE BOOK

The *Quality Handbook for Health Care Organizations* is organized according to topic, with theoretical issues outlined and practical tools explained in each chapter. At the end of each chapter, sections titled "Things to Think About" offer questions designed to personalize the material in the chapter in keeping with our goal of enabling a manager to use the information to best advantage on the job. Managers may find the final questions useful as exercises for training staff in principles of quality management as well. For students of quality management or any other health services occupation, the concluding exercises provide a review of the significant ideas outlined in each chapter.

Our approach is a functional one. We hope to provide a useful on-the-job training manual as well as a resource for the how-to questions that arise during the normal working day. In the following chapters, we stress procedures and methods for department heads, managers, supervisors—all those health care leaders who are close to bedside care and who influence the delivery of services to patients—to assess the care they deliver through collecting and analyzing quality data. We discuss criteria for prioritization of performance improvement efforts and for resource allocation, keeping in mind the delicate balancing act that managers must perform among clinical services, human resources requirements, budgetary restrictions, risk management and legal issues, patient satisfaction, health outcomes, and serious incidents or events.

Using hypothetical case studies compiled from our experience to illustrate significant themes, we offer examples of problem-solving techniques and discuss how to implement performance improvements using the Plan-Do-Check-Act (PDCA) methodology. Our central message concerns the power of data—for evaluating care, establishing best practices, and developing guidelines for your unit or service. Through the quality management framework, we illustrate how to establish accountability and better communication among staff and throughout the organization—and, what is most important, how quality management techniques can lead to better outcomes for your patients.

In Chapter One, we discuss the role of the manager and the many pressures confronting the manager in the provision of care in today's complex health care environment. This role is defined not only by the institution but by the government and through regulatory agencies. Quality management methodology helps managers better define and understand their responsibilities.

Chapter Two briefly sketches the history of quality management methods and traces how quality principles have evolved through the decades to have an important impact on the way health care services are delivered and understood today both by the public and by the health care organization. Since the manager is the person primarily responsible for establishing a quality management framework on a given unit, and for providing the public, the regulatory agencies, the bedside worker, the administration of the hospital, and the patient with quality information, the manager should be familiar with the basic principles and tools.

Chapter Three begins a discussion of how to develop quality data for evaluating care, highlighting how criteria should conform to pre-identified goals. Once data elements are defined and collected, data can be used to assess present practices and to establish targets for performance improvements. As managers must work within budgetary restrictions, they have to make choices regarding where to use resources. We offer a tool for prioritization of improvements, based on providing the best outcomes for the greatest number of people.

Chapter Four continues the discussion of quality data and measurements, including issues involved in carefully defining and developing appropriate quality indicators to evaluate and monitor services. Once quality indicators are defined, databases can be compiled to review the interrelationships among different aspects of care. The goal of data analysis is to understand the care being delivered and to identify opportunities for improvements through objective information. Data must be interpreted and communicated to be effective, and this chapter suggests the complex interrelationships among caregivers who collaborate for improved patient services.

Chapter Five outlines the basic statistical tools and techniques used in quality management data analysis, which we offer so that managers can understand the range and variability of the information they collect and interpret how that information reflects the care being delivered on their unit or service. From cause-and-effect diagrams to standard deviation, the discussion centers on how a manager can use these tools to improve patient care. As communication is all-important, this chapter offers examples of different ways to display data for maximum effect.

Chapter Six explains how data provide the basis for performance improvement, whether of existing processes, in the development of new ones, or as a response to an adverse event or incident. Proactive improvements, sparked by near-miss data and a culture of open communication, help prevent incidents and eliminate or reduce risk to patients. Using the PDCA cycle for evaluating processes and for establishing criteria for improvement, the manager can implement new processes and procedures while involving the multidisciplinary team in improvement efforts.

Chapter Seven illustrates the advantages of using clinical pathways and guidelines as tools for standardizing care and eliminating unwarranted variation in care. Using guidelines promotes coordination of the delivery of multiple services and enhances communication about the progress of care as the patient moves throughout the continuum. Guidelines also provide invaluable information for how to manage a crisis. Measuring whether or not the standard of care was met, through variance data, enables the manager to determine which patients did not receive the appropriate interventions and which interventions did not result in the expected outcomes. These measures help the manager organize the workload on the unit, improve patient care, inform the multidisciplinary team about any gaps in that care, and anticipate length of stay.

Chapter Eight describes how information is transferred from the bedside throughout the managerial hierarchy to the Board of Trustees and back again to influence improved care practices. It also addresses issues involved in accountability. Through an example of how the NS-LIJHS established a sophisticated and all-encompassing committee structure, we illustrate the advantages of a strong communication framework to coordinate and implement improvements throughout a hospital or health care system.

Chapter Nine outlines how to use quality management methods to address serious events or incidents, to correct flaws in the process of care, and to minimize risks to patient safety. Analytic tools such as root cause analysis and failure mode effects and analysis are presented. Examples of various types of errors and improvement efforts are offered to suggest how to manage in the case of a crisis. Communication, collaboration, data, and commitment all contribute to lessening the devastating effects of an adverse or sentinel event.

Chapter Ten gives examples of how various departments within a health system use quality management methods to assess and improve care in a collaborative fashion. Because the delivery of excellent patient care requires multidisciplinary involvement and communication among different disciplines, these examples are designed to illustrate the pervasive and unifying theme of quality, how quality information crosses departments and services and can be used to better understand the intricate interrelationships of providing care in a complex health care environment.

The handbook concludes with a review of the major themes and a discussion of how to use benchmarks to develop best practices for your service. The goal throughout is to provide practical and realistic methods and tools to promote superior management.

TOWARD A COMMON GOAL

Our goal is to share this vision, especially with people responsible for preserving patient safety, minimizing risks to patients, and maintaining high standards of quality services in today's increasingly complex world of health care delivery. Much of this responsibility sits squarely on managers' shoulders—all managers, not only clinical managers or senior managers but all those who supervise departments, work with staff, and have an impact on patient care.

Our experience has taught us that when managers and department leaders are offered the tools to improve the care they deliver, they grab them enthusiastically—and make good use of them. We have been reaching out and teaching managers the tools, methods, techniques, and philosophy of quality management, based on our daily experience with bedside care, with great success.

This book incorporates what we have learned from our students as well as our experience and expertise in quality management. Our intention is to provide more than theory: we offer theory combined with the skills and information required to assess, evaluate, analyze, improve, and communicate about the delivery of care. Others involved in health care services, such as administrators, senior leadership, and policymakers who shape health care, will benefit by understanding today's science of quality as well. There is no more worthwhile endeavor than providing vulnerable people with excellent and compassionate care. It is our hope that this handbook offers those interested in health care the tools to reach this goal.

ACKNOWLEDGMENTS

This book could not have been written without the encouragement and support of many people. Chief among them, we would like to thank the CEO and president of the NS-LIJHS, Michael J. Dowling, for his commitment to quality. We owe a debt of gratitude to the many dedicated professionals who have worked with us to define quality. And to our families, who have encouraged us in this enterprise with love and patience, and believed in its importance, we owe our understanding of what it means to care. Doris, Richard, and Bob—we thank you.

Special thanks to our talented graphic designers and illustrators, Rico Rosales and Hillel Dlugacz.

Great Neck, New York   Yosef D. Dlugacz
January 2004   Andrea Restifo
                                                              Alice Greenwood

⟞ The Authors

Yosef D. Dlugacz, Ph.D., senior vice president of quality management for the North Shore–Long Island Jewish Health System, is responsible for oversight of the extensive quality management program, which spans a broad spectrum of services provided by eighteen health care facilities. His responsibility extends to developing sophisticated methodologies for performance improvement, targeting initiatives based on focused data analyses, and communicating information about improvement processes and procedures via a complex quality committee structure that he has developed and implemented throughout the system.

Other supervisory duties include utilization management programs, analyses of incidents and sentinel events, responsibility for communicating regulatory requirements to hospital facilities, directing quality research, and maintaining quality across the continuum of care. He has lectured extensively, nationally and internationally, and is the author of numerous professional articles. He has consulted on quality management throughout the United States, Europe, the Middle East, and China. He is adjunct research professor at New York University and has been appointed visiting professor to Beijing University's MBA program. He is also a guest lecturer at Helsingborg Hospital and Uppsala University in Sweden.

Andrea Restifo, R.N., M.P.A, is vice president of quality management for the North Shore–Long Island Jewish Health System. She is responsible for the operations of the system's Quality Management Department, facilitating all quality management activities at the multiple sites. Restifo, a fifteen-year veteran of the system, coordinates all quality management reports to the Board of Trustees and develops internal quality documents, appropriate to each venue, for distribution throughout the system. She has participated in developing standardized measurements for quality indicators and ensures that the educational methodology is communicated effectively across the system. She has collaborated on instructional materials for performance improvement that have been presented at numerous national and international health care conferences. She received her undergraduate BSN degree at Villanova University, Pennsylvania, and was awarded a Nursing Distinction Award. She received her Master's of Public Administration at Long Island University, New York, graduating with honors. She is a member of the National Association for Healthcare Quality, earning her Certified Professional in Healthcare Quality (CPHQ) in 1997. She is also a member of the New York Association for Healthcare Quality, Inc., and is a Villanova Nursing alumna.

Alice Greenwood received her Ph.D. in linguistics with a specialization in communication styles of different social groups. She has published numerous scholarly articles on linguistics, language and gender, and child witness testimony. Her scientific research in discourse analysis was conducted at Bell Labs and AT&T Labs in New Jersey, where she was a communications and information analyst. While there, Greenwood coauthored a book on the acoustics of American speech sounds. She has worked as a writer and editor for numerous popular books, including the biography of President Clinton's surgeon general nominee, Dr. Henry Foster, and a prenatal care book for low-literate women that was sponsored by the What to Expect Foundation. As an information and research specialist for the North Shore–Long Island Jewish Health Systems Quality Management Department (probably the only Quality Management Department in the country with an academic linguist on staff), she has helped the department publish its successes in peer-reviewed journals and was instrumental in developing the application for the Pinnacle Award, for which the system received Honorable Mention. She teaches the communication modules for the quality management course for managers and has most recently been made faculty at the Academy of the National Center for the Prosecution of Child Abuse (NCPCA).

Lawrence Scherr, M.D., MACP, is the Betsey Cushing Whitney Dean as well as senior vice president, academic affairs, for the North Shore–Long Island Jewish Health System. He also directs the Community Health and Public Policy Program for NS-LIJHS and chairs the Ethics Committee of North Shore University Hospital. From 1967 to 2001, he was chairman of the Department of Medicine, North Shore University Hospital. He is a professor of medicine, first at Cornell University Medical College and currently at New York University School of Medicine.

Scherr is master and chairman emeritus of the Board of Governors and the Board of Regents, president and president emeritus of the American College of Physicians; a past officer of the American Board of Internal Medicine and the American Board of Medical Specialties; chairman, Accreditation Council for Graduate Medical Education and chairman of the Residency Review Committee in Internal Medicine. He also served on the New York State Health Commissioner's Task Force on Health Reform as well as the Association of American Medical Colleges' Committee on Health Care Reform. He was chairman of the New York State Board for Medicine and chairman of the New York State Council on Graduate Medical Education. He served with President Clinton's White House Review Group on health care reform as well as on numerous other national committees involving ethics, health policy, medical practice and strategic planning for health care, graduate medical education, physician manpower, and efficacy of clinical practice.

The Quality Handbook for Health Care Organizations

CHAPTER ONE

The Role of the Manager

Imagine yourself on the first day of your new job. Where do you start? Regardless of whether you manage a unit such as Oncology, a process such as infection control, or a service such as Pharmacy or Nutrition, more than likely you have a staff, a budget, and your own manager to whom you report. You are responsible for the smooth operation of a specific environment, one with a defined scope of care. You may have a set of expectations and responsibilities that are not very clearly delineated, those that your manager or supervisor expects of you, and those that you expect of yourself and of your staff.

Before you can get your coat off and pick up a pencil, a problem erupts. This is health care, and crises are a daily and anticipated event. What approach do you take to handling the problem? Your reaction and the procedures you use are important, as your staff will take their cue from you for how to behave in a crisis. Rest assured that problem solving, quick decision making, and crisis management will be among your primary tasks as a manager.

SERVING THE ORGANIZATION

Perhaps it was once possible to confine your work solely to your own unit, but today most health care managers and supervisors are required to interact with many people and departments outside their unit, all of whom have their individual agendas, philosophies, techniques, and expectations. Managers have to develop a host of working relationships and achieve some sort of balance between their own expectations and responsibilities and those of the rest of the organization. For instance, hospital administrators are concerned about financial issues and reimbursement and will demand that you work within a budget to provide efficient and effective services. Managers from various departments—Legal, Planning, Materials, Environment, Risk Management, or Human Resources—may ask you for information or may invite you or members of your staff to collaborate on projects. And your own manager or supervisor may request reports about your decisions and monitor how you deliver care.

Physicians also require that you manage your responsibilities as effectively as possible so that their patients' needs and expectations are well met. Without an amiable working relationship with the physicians who admit patients and have the primary responsibility for their medical care, your job becomes much more difficult.

And there's more. The manager has to be familiar with and work in a manner that is congruent with the organization's articulated mission and vision. A good health system will actually demand that its guiding principles be incorporated into the daily work of the staff and reflected in the services delivered to the patients. Also, most health facilities prepare a strategic plan that outlines their goals for the future and that dictates how resources will be allocated. The managers must all know their own roles in the strategic plan, and not solely in terms of what the plan entails. Managers actually help shape the plan because goals need to be identified and objectives delineated. The strategic plan articulates a sense of direction for the managers, one that can be used to effectively encourage staff to meet expectations. Figure 1.1 illustrates the many internal and external forces that you must respond to as a manager, while managing the staff, budget, environment, and clinical services of your own department.

Serving the Patient

The manager, then, has to handle crises, juggle competing agendas, administer and provide efficient and effective services, manage staff

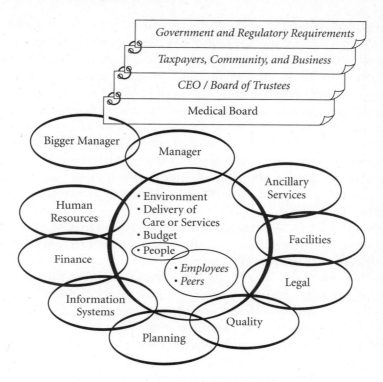

Government and Regulatory Requirements

Taxpayers, Community, and Business

CEO / Board of Trustees

Medical Board

Bigger Manager

Manager

Ancillary Services

Human Resources

• Environment
• Delivery of
  Care or Services
• Budget
• People

Facilities

Finance

• Employees
• Peers

Legal

Information Systems

Quality

Planning

Figure 1.1.   The Complex Role of the Manager.

schedules, competency, and workloads, and do so within a restricted budget in addition to being accountable to the organization's administrative and medical hierarchy—all the while maintaining the all-important role of being the patients' advocate. It is the manager who mediates between direct beside care to people who are vulnerable, unhappy, and often out of control of their lives and the rest of the complex health care organization.

To manage bedside care and direct staff effectively, the manager must be organized and gather the information required to set daily priorities to ensure the proper flow of activities that will enhance patient care. Morning rounds as shifts change, for example, are a good opportunity to acquire knowledge about the patients and their needs in order to set the activities of the day in motion. Staff input, together with predefined expectations and goals, influence priorities for providing services to the patients.

Patients today, unlike the patients of decades past, feel entitled to the highest quality of care—and they are educated about the relationship between medical interventions and changes in clinical status. They expect interventions that will improve the way they feel, and if they are not feeling better, they want to know why. Also, as patients are accountable for their bills, they scrutinize the tests they receive and evaluate the interventions and the physician contact in terms of effectiveness. This appraisal of the exchange of goods and services for improved outcomes transforms the traditional relationship between patient and caregiver from one of physical and emotional dependency to a more rational and equal role paralleling that of a consumer and a provider.

As a result, today's managers must understand that the patient is an active consumer of health care services rather than a passive and compliant responder, and they are responsible for training their staff accordingly. Patient satisfaction can influence the organization's budget and thus indirectly the manager's own position. Simply stated, without patients, you have no one to work for. Not only must there be adequate patient census for the manager's services to be evaluated positively, the services must be of excellent quality as well. If many patients complain that the staffing on the manager's service was inadequate, or that care was poorly delivered, or that errors occurred, or that the equipment or environment was not excellent or functioning properly, the manager hears about it. This is as it should be. Health care should serve the patient.

Patients expect that their care should be respectful, courteous, polite, considerate, and compassionate; managers are accountable for providing patients with appropriate education—about their care, their hospital stay, their disease process, and expectations for posthospital care. Patients need to understand informed consent forms, discharge plans, and medication regimens; they may also need orientation to hospital services, pain management, patient and consumer rights, and medical procedures.

Patients demand and expect efficient and effective care, care that eliminates or reduces their problem without incurring undue expense from the inappropriate use of resources. Understandably, patients have no desire to pay for unnecessary services or for a prolonged hospital stay that their insurance carrier won't cover. As paying customers, they introduce a new voice into the chorus of health care services, one that forces the manager to balance all their requirements, their needs as patients and also as intelligent consumers. Therefore, the manager needs to coordinate staff for appropriate patient services while attending to the patients' physical environment as well as their emotional needs and social expectations. It is never good business to have unsatisfied customers.

In a service business whose consumers are emotionally and physically compromised, care is often rendered not because of direct payment expectations but simply because it is the right thing to do. Many hospitals have as part of their mission that they provide care to everyone, regardless of ability to pay. This decency puts a burden on the managers to manage especially wisely, so as to balance good patient care with the financial responsibilities of the organization. If a patient receives a letter stating that henceforth all hospital expenses will no longer be paid by the insurance carrier but by the patient, the manager and the care provider have to determine how best to continue to manage that patient's care. There may be choices that would satisfy the monetary constraints of the patient without compromising good care. For example, the manager or caregiver could provide extensive education to the patient regarding discharge expectations or provide follow-up care in a less acute facility.

Serving the Public

People realize that one day they or someone they love might become a patient in a health care facility; therefore, it is unsurprising that the public demands that health care facilities deliver outstanding care. Health care is expected to be responsive to the needs of the community, with community representatives, who form the Board of Trustees, charged with ensuring that care is appropriate and safe, and that it meets the expectations of the local population. The manager of a unit or service answers to the Board, directly or indirectly, about the delivery of care.

Various monitoring agencies including the state and federal health departments and regulatory agencies such as the Joint Commission for the Accreditation of Healthcare Organizations (JCAHO), also representing the concerns of the public, have a big impact on how services are delivered. Today's manager is expected to be compliant with regulations.

Compliance, however, is merely the beginning of effective management. Regulations should be considered as a kind of compass designed to supply direction for advancing patient care and improving the workings of the unit or service. For example, the requirement to provide patients with a safe environment details how to do it, when to do it, why, and how often. Although creating a safe environment might involve expenses that should be budgeted, in terms of personnel, equipment, and efficient processes, ignoring the requirement or merely giving compliance minimal lip service could lead to problems, unsatisfied customers, unhappy administrators, and a displeased Board of Trustees. The purpose of the regulation is to encourage health care facilities to do the right thing for their patients, regardless of expense.

The general public has a big impact on health care services also. The public perception of care, especially of poor care, influences the financial success of health care facilities. Information regarding quality and safety in health care, and about specific hospitals, physicians, and medical services, is becoming readily available through the Internet and the media. No one wants inadequate or inappropriate care; no one wants to enter a hospital with a reputation for endangering patients. No hospital wants the care it delivers to be labeled as substandard. It is part of the manager's job to ensure that the hospital has a good reputation and is highly regarded in the public eye.

Media attention has focused on the mistakes, errors, problems, and flaws in today's health care environment. The widely discussed 1999 Institute of Medicine report, *To Err Is Human,* condemns health care delivery in this country as inadequate, inefficient, fragmented, unscientific, and in need of fundamental change. Private organizations including the Leapfrog Group and the Midwest Business Group have taken it upon themselves to dictate standards for quality care, insisting on accountability from hospitals.

These groups have a great deal of buying power and they want to be assured that their money is well spent. The *Wall Street Journal* reported that "poor quality care costs companies around $1,700 to $2,000 per covered employee a year" (Landers, 2002). Indeed, these groups require proof of good management and good quality—the two go hand in hand—and are outcome-oriented. Patients can exercise the privilege of going where they think the best care is offered, and large businesses can negotiate contracts for their employees where they think they will get the best results. Poor health care quality costs money.

Public expectations pressure health care institutions to provide—and to be able to document—safe quality care. Managers are therefore concerned not to make mistakes, to monitor safe practices whatever the scope of their charge, and to be able to rationalize and defend the processes and decisions they make as being beneficial to the patient and the health care institution.

Managers, then, have to provide excellent clinical service while keeping their eye on the financial aspects of the delivery of care as well. A busy unit does not necessarily reflect a cost-effective unit that is providing good clinical care to its patients. A busy unit may simply be a poorly managed unit, one that serves neither the patients nor the institution well. For example, inefficiencies in bed turnover can keep the beds full but actually mask the fact that new patients are not coming into the unit and therefore revenue is lost, and worst of all, that patients are inappropriately cared for. To equalize the pressures between financial success and excellent clinical outcomes requires that the manager work with the managers of other departments (such as Housekeeping, Discharge Planning, and Social Work) to efficiently move each patient through the continuum of care.

GETTING HELP FROM ALL THE RIGHT PLACES

How can a manager begin to juggle all these responsibilities, and to acquire the skills necessary to manage all that needs to be managed?

Enter the government.

Health care today is a highly regulated industry. The regulations are designed to assist health care leaders and managers as well as to protect the patient and monitor the delivery of care. This is as it should be, because a health care institution is, in many ways, unique. What other kind of organization deals with the *business* of life and death, pain and suffering, illness and well-being? Or with social issues such as undocumented residents who are afraid of the bureaucracy of the admissions process and use Emergency Departments as primary care physicians for their children, and who often can't pay for services, or the elderly, who have no place to go upon discharge and who also often can't pay for services. Social issues. Financial issues. And, of course, complicated medical issues. Health care is a business that needs very careful management.

If you drive along a small, untraveled country lane, you would resent a series of traffic lights that attempted to control the nonexistent congestion. However, when you drive on chaotic, overcrowded roads that converge at busy intersections, you are grateful for the control imposed by traffic lights. In addition to being useful and appropriate, the lights are effective because laws dictate that drivers react appropriately to them, and drivers honor the rules out of a mixture of agreement with their purpose and fear of the consequences of breaking them.

Regulatory Agencies Help Define Good Care

The numerous, lengthy, and complex government regulations for health care institutions became necessary because care was chaotic, and the public had the accompanying fear of accidents. Hospitals were not being managed well, nor were they managing their responsibilities adequately. Patients were not receiving standardized care; hospitals were increasingly unsuccessful as financial organizations, incurring massive debts with profoundly unsatisfied customers. Performance requirements had little standardization, and the institutions had few formal operating principles to follow.

Confusion reigned even about what kind of service a hospital should be in the business of providing. It was not universally apparent what it meant to provide good care. Should care be based on principles related to financial reimbursement? If so, then delivering good care and managing services effectively involved understanding severity indices, the acuity of illness, and appropriate diagnoses—the bases of reimbursement. Or perhaps good care should be based on competition for public regard (as in, mine is better than yours), in which case quality indicators such as mortality and morbidity rates would be the central focus.

In an attempt to stem the confusion, to ensure parity for services, and to protect patients from harm, today the management of health care services is carefully regulated—how it is delivered, when it is delivered, in what environment it is delivered, to whom it is delivered, and with what outcome. The JCAHO, the Department of Health (DOH) in each state, and many other regulatory agencies require health care organizations to define the structure, the processes, and the staff necessary to manage the delivery of quality care.

Overall, these regulatory and oversight agencies force organizations to examine the competency of their staff and to evaluate the quality of the care they deliver in order to assess whether or not they are doing a good job. Good care is now equated with quality care—care that is measurably safe, of the highest standard, evidence-based, uniformly delivered, with the appropriate utilization of resources and services.

The JCAHO expects processes to be developed, implemented, monitored, and assessed on an ongoing basis, and it is the managers' responsibility to comply with these expectations.

During the accreditation survey process, surveyors interact with unit managers, inquiring about the process and provision of care and about performance improvement efforts that each manager has introduced and supervised. Surveyors also interview staff and patients on the unit to verify that the staff has been properly educated and is competent (another managerial responsibility) and that the patients express satisfaction with their care. And the JCAHO is only one agency to which the manager is accountable.

State health departments can take a different focus. In New York State, the DOH evaluates outcomes of care in addition to evaluating the processes used to deliver that care. It monitors mortality for high-risk procedures (such as cardiac surgery), incidents and errors, and patient complaints—and reports its findings out publicly. Good care is defined as having successful results for the patients.

Regulatory Agencies Help Define the Manager's Role

These regulatory agencies also provide additional definition about the manager's role in the organization, regardless of department, and set expectations about management responsibilities. Before the regulatory agencies began setting standards, managers had very few, if any, guidelines for what was expected of them in their role. Hospital administrators and human resource professionals had no principled basis on which to hire professional staff because they had no established criteria for good management.

Before the oversight of regulatory agencies, administrators would rely on the managers themselves to define their own roles within the organization and to develop their personal set of responsibilities. Administrators had little experience with the kinds of professional expertise their managers had (nursing, pharmacy, respiratory therapy, social work, and so on), and therefore they were at a disadvantage in attempting to direct their delivery of quality services or evaluating their performance.

Now, based on JCAHO criteria, Human Resource departments have a prescribed methodology for staffing that can actually identify for administrators the appropriate qualifications and requirements for a manager. For example, the JCAHO standards for leadership specifically include department heads, managers, and supervisors, and outline for managers their scope of responsibilities: to plan, direct, coordinate, integrate, provide, and improve health care services that are cost-effective, responsive to member and community needs, congruent with the mission and vision or the organization, and designed to improve health outcomes. Piece of cake, right? And these are just a few of many such managerial responsibilities. Managers, in other words, are expected to do the right thing for the right reason and do it well. Furthermore, managers are expected to measure the care they deliver and present that information to the governing board of the institution.

Regulatory Agencies Help Define the Manager's Responsibilities

JCAHO standards also outline the structures and processes for how this is supposed to happen. Department leaders, to be effective, are expected to integrate and coordinate departmental services with the hospital's primary functions and with other departments; to develop and implement appropriate policies and procedures; to make recommendations about staffing needs and qualifications; to continually assess and improve departmental performance; to maintain appropriate quality control programs; to provide for orientation, in-service training, and continuing education of everyone on their staff; and to recommend space and other resources needed by the department. These responsibilities have to be met or the organization will not be fully accredited.

Moreover, managers are also required to document that these responsibilities have been met. And not only to document appropriately but to communicate effectively. The JCAHO defines different layers of communication within the health care hierarchy. Managers are expected to communicate with their own staff and employees, and also to their managers, the administrators, and the medical boards. The JCAHO even sets expectations about what kinds of information the managers should require of their staff and service providers.

GETTING THE NECESSARY TOOLS FOR THE JOB

All these regulations and recommendations make the managers' job easier, their role clearer, and their expectations better articulated. But what a huge task! Without a deliberate process for handling the responsibilities of the job, managers can easily find themselves overwhelmed.

How would you, as a manager, go about assessing and improving your department's performance? Would you know where to start? The JCAHO requires that you improve performance using data, and that you identify, gather, and analyze data, both internally and in collaboration with other departments. Most managers have no background or education that would enable them to easily respond to this mandate.

Data collection is required for budgetary reasons and to help Human Resources allocate appropriate staff for the delivery of required services. Data are necessary for quality control in Pharmacy, in the laboratories, in radiology, and for the blood bank, to name a few examples. Even more than using data to meet regulatory expectations, data can be used to measure care in order to evaluate and improve services. How do you know what kinds of data to collect, or how to collect information so that it is reliable or how to analyze data for performance improvement?

Enter quality management.

Quality Management to the Rescue

It is the hospital's or health system's Quality Management Department that has the responsibility for interpreting the regulatory standards for hospital accreditation and for helping managers design programs tailored to the specific requirements of their particular service. By explaining the expectations of the regulatory agencies in terms of developing appropriate measurements for evaluating care, quality management methods actually help managers determine what type of data they should collect, how it should be collected, and how to analyze it to improve the processes for which they are accountable.

One of the basic tenets of quality management is that objective information, in the form of data, can be used to assess and improve performance, providing managers with the building blocks they need to construct a well-run department or service. With the proper data, a manager can evaluate the delivery of service and set goals and expectations for improvement. (There is always room for improvement.) Not only can quality management data be used to help managers meet their evaluative and assessment goals, and to motivate staff behavior, the data can also identify problems for proactive improvement efforts. Managers need to know what the problems are before they can begin correcting them.

No Need to Reinvent the Wheel

Using a consistent quality management methodology allows managers to develop processes that can be generalized across multiple issues. This is very productive—you don't want to respond on an ad hoc basis to every problem that arises, hoping to reinvent the wheel under the pressure of a crisis. Moreover, having a defined methodology helps you inform and educate your staff about your expectations—things are to be done in a certain deliberate and sensible way and not another.

The methodology that we use in our Health System, Plan-Do-Check-Act (PDCA), developed by the quality thinkers W. A. Shewhart and W. Edwards Deming in the 1920s, prescribes asking questions, collecting relevant data, planning an action or intervention, then implementing the action and finally assessing the effectiveness of the action. This quality management methodology enables a focused and informed response to the evaluation and improvement of processes, so that managers are well prepared to handle the unexpected, which they can expect to crop up daily.

Ask and Ye Shall Receive

Depending on what kind of manager you are, and what you manage, whether it be a service (Social Work) or a unit (Nursing) or a process (Risk Management, Infection Control), you need to ask appropriate questions about the daily functioning of your department in order to understand your delivery of care. You may want information about staffing levels and competency, about the environment of care and the clinical issues facing your patients. You may need to coordinate with other disciplines to provide your patients with effective services.

For example, as a nurse manager, you might begin with asking this series of questions: What kind of unit is this? Who are the patients? What are their clinical and social issues? What would be the ideal way to run such a unit? What expertise is necessary for staff? What are anticipatable problems? To answer these kinds of questions, a nurse manager needs to collect data regarding the number of patients on the unit (that is, take a simple census), the type of diagnoses they have, and the services required for patients with those diagnoses to receive good care. With the resulting data, the manager can determine what kind of resources are required for effective management of the unit— appropriate staffing, competency requirements of the staff, anticipated bed use, length of stay predictions for the delivery of effective care, anticipated turnaround time, and what could be identified as appropriate and successful outcomes. The data that these questions elicit can make the manager's job more coherent and the unit and staff easier to manage.

Another example: If your unit is responsible for elderly patients with pneumonia, collecting comparative data, which quality management supplies to managers, would alert you that such patients are at greater risk for falls and pressure injuries than other patients, and that their nutritional requirements might be critical to maintain health. An awareness of these risks will give you the ammunition, in the form of hard data, to ask for the resources to develop a fall-prevention program or to acquire specialty beds to avoid skin ulcers. You might also develop an educational program for staff regarding fall safety, and for the assessment and treatment of pressure injuries. A patient fall can result in a great expenditure of resources; prevention is always the better way. Avoiding risks and adverse events is key to successful management.

The Blueprint for Success

But complying with regulations, collecting data, and using a consistent methodology for the evaluation and improvement of processes and performance are only the starting points for a good manager. Managers also need a philosophy if they are to function effectively and provide direction for their employees. If the employees know that their manager is operating within a specified framework—in the language of the JCAHO, doing something right for the right reason—they can more productively do their own jobs because their managers are providing them with guidance and a rationale for what they do. Within a specific framework, every incident, problem, or process is handled with a structure, rather than on a case-by-case or crisis-by-crisis basis. Furthermore, if you use data as the basis of decisions, then everyone on your staff knows that decisions are based on objective criteria rather than subjective impressions or capricious or random impulses. Grounding decisions in data offers staff a useful reference point for how to behave.

Quality management provides the health care manager with a working philosophy, one that focuses on the processes of delivering services the right way for the right reasons at the right time. Quality management specialists have developed the tools, techniques, and expertise to measure the processes and to plan for improvement, and quality management methodology can help managers develop reasonable expectations about clinical outcomes. In other words, working within a quality management framework, managers have a deliberate approach to care so that their staff will understand where they are coming from—and, more important, going to. Figure 1.2 illustrates how the quality management program provides the foundation for the manager and staff to develop consistently defined measurements for assessing and improving care.

Based on the information revealed through quality management measures, improvement initiatives can be planned and developed that are consistent with the strategic plan, the vision, and the mission of the health care institution. Our experience in the eighteen-hospital North Shore–Long Island Jewish Health System (NS-LIJHS) has taught us how integrating quality management into every facet of the organization can implement positive change and improved performance. We do much more than ensure compliance with regulations; that is merely a jumping-off point for monitoring care. Our health system is as successful as it is—in the year 2002 alone, the system received a JCAHO score of 99, one of our hospitals was rated the "best hospital in the country" by an independent survey, two of our hospitals were

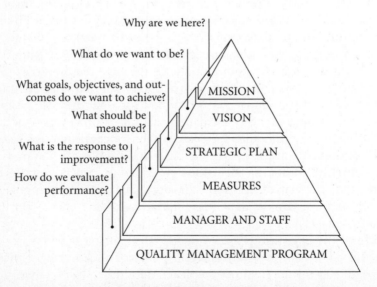

Figure 1.2.   Building Blocks for a Quality Organization.

awarded the prestigious Magnet nursing award, among many other honors and tributes, and in 1999 the system received the prestigious Codman Award for innovations in outcomes measurements—because quality is embedded into the processes and structures that cross the organization and the entire continuum of care.

Our leadership, including the managers of departments, is committed to weaving a culture of quality into every piece of the organization. Principles of quality management are presented to new employees during orientation. Managers from every discipline attend a two-day course on quality management methodologies and performance improvement strategies to increase their skills on their units and to ensure that they have the necessary tools to do their jobs well while balancing quality, safety, budget, and competency issues. There is no need to wait for administrators or other supervisors to inform managers that patient safety and excellent care is their own responsibility. Working within a quality management framework, managers can establish accountability and better communication with staff while delivering better outcomes for patients.

SUMMARY

The health care manager is expected to take care of all of these responsibilities:

- Provide efficient and effective services in the delivery of care.
- Balance competing agendas of other departments and services within the organization.
- Manage staff schedules.
- Work within a budget.
- Educate patients about their care and hospitalization.
- Respond to the mission and vision of the organization.
- Understand and comply with government regulations.
- Maintain appropriate quality control programs.
- Supervise training and education of the staff.
- Use data to improve performance.
- Work within a quality management framework.
- Define a philosophy for the delivery of care.

Things to Think About:

- You are given the responsibility to teach and train new managers, regardless of service or unit, to do their job.

    What criteria would you use to evaluate their performance?

    What training do you think would be most valuable?

    What information do they need to best perform their job?

    How would you handle the role of regulatory requirements?

    What would you tell them about data?

    What advice would you give a new manager?

CHAPTER TWO

Managing Quality

A s a manager, you want to be successful and assure your patients and administration that you are delivering quality care. But what exactly does the concept of *quality* in health care mean, and why is it important for you to define the concept for yourself and your staff? Regulatory agencies attempt to define quality through mandated standards and the use of comparative measures. Hospital administrators may understand quality in terms of maximum reimbursement and appropriate utilization—getting the biggest bang for the buck. Physicians and nurses may define quality still differently, with physicians focusing on interventions and therapeutic success while nurses focus on the immediate environment, measuring quality in terms of falls, restraint use, skin care, complaints and satisfaction, and psychosocial issues.

DEFINING QUALITY

Struggling to define the idea of quality may seem an unnecessary endeavor to many physicians, who understand quality care as the result of being well trained, educated, competent, and experienced—a kind of tautology: "I am qualified to give good care; therefore the care I give is good." If the outcomes of care are unsuccessful, as when a patient dies, such a physician might say that the fault lies with the illness; the patient was too sick to be cured. Maybe so, maybe not. In any case, degree of illness is an unsatisfactory way to think about quality because it allows no accountability or room for assessment for improvement.

For doctors who deal with physiological factors (such as tumors or blood levels), quality might be related to how the disease is progressing. But do patients evaluate quality the same way? More likely, patients define quality care in terms of how they feel and how soon, if ever, they can resume their normal lives. Quality, then, must maintain a balance between what doctors do and how patients feel.

Even though the definition of quality in health care has changed over the years, as care has become more complex and a greater number of people and processes become involved in the delivery of care, some fundamentals remain unchanged. Patients are basically helpless and trust their doctors and other professional staff to take good care of them. Since the manager's job is to mediate among the organization, the physician, and the patient, the manager has a tremendous role in determining the quality of care delivered. Our quality philosophy is based on the very simple notion that the patient always comes first— simple as an idea, perhaps, but quite complicated to operationalize.

For the Manager

Although quality is a difficult and slippery concept, it is important to nail it down because managing quality, in a sense, is what all managers have to do. As a manager, you want to have a concrete definition or standard of quality care that can be objectively assessed and communicated to your staff. The definition should be broad enough to span many processes and provide a commonality whether delivering care at the bedside on a unit, day or night, or in the operating room, or providing technical support in the laboratory or the pharmacy, in the Emergency Department, or with services such as Housekeeping, Nutrition, Home Care, or Materials, to suggest just a few areas. In other words, quality care is about a process and a mindset rather than a series of actions or responsibilities. The more dynamic your definition, the more useful it will be to you.

Where does the patient fit into your definition of quality? Patients, as consumers of health care services, are quite different from the kinds of consumers who visit Disneyland for a good time and evaluate the quality of their experience in terms of the cleanliness of their hotels and the waiting times on line. Consumers of health care services do not come to a hospital for entertainment and pleasure; their satisfaction is related to other criteria. Patients evaluate the quality of their care based on the impact health care interventions have made on their illness, or matched their expectations, or improved the quality of their lives.

For the Patient

It is important to remember that patients are not all alike. Their perceptions of the quality of their care are based on their social and emotional state as well as their physiological response to treatment. They don't constitute a homogeneous group that can be easily and uniformly satisfied. Rather, they are a collection of highly individual and complex traits. If meeting patients' expectations should be incorporated into the manager's definition of quality, which patients are we talking about? Surveys reveal that satisfaction rates differ depending on the reason and the time patients are hospitalized. In the same institution, patients in labor and delivery can be highly satisfied while patients on oncology units or with chronic disease are not. This seems obvious, but nonetheless should be remembered when thinking about patient satisfaction. Your definition of quality should be able to accommodate the needs of all patients, without regard to why they are in the hospital.

You will find some similarities among patient expectations, however. All patients want to be treated with dignity and compassion, and to have their privacy respected and their individuality honored. But even the seemingly simple things, such as responding to call-bells quickly, may involve more than a superficial response.

For the Institution

The call-bells have to work properly (which may involve Engineering) and be positioned so that the patients can reach them (Housekeeping). The patients should understand how to use them and under what circumstances (Patient Education). When a patient uses the call-bell, someone should respond (staffing ratios and nursing education). The manager of a patient care unit needs to supervise all these processes and staff and interact with these other departments to deliver quality care.

If response to the call-bells is slow, the consequences can be serious, leading to adverse events and incidents. A patient who does not get a timely response (according to the patient, not the nurse) may attempt to get out of bed and fall. The fall may result in a fracture or require surgery. The manager then is held responsible and is expected to supply information about what caused the incident, and to make corrections so that it doesn't happen again. It's far better to have processes in place that reduce problems than to wait and respond to problems as they occur. As manager, you must evaluate the processes of care with an eye to establishing processes that prevent adverse occurrences.

If you manage a Pharmacy or a Radiology or Social Services Department, you are responsible for similar seemingly simple processes that generally are not so simple to manage at all. No patient wants to be kept waiting, either in a hallway because an MRI schedule got backed up or for medication because the computers are down in the pharmacy. How do you resolve these problems? How many people and processes are involved? Patients want to go home when they are released, not be forced to wait for lack of transport staff or completed discharge instructions. Your responsibilities might include managing these processes also. The definition of providing quality care should be broad enough to encompass any and all of these circumstances. Again, quality is about providing the best care for the patient, and about developing the processes and measurements that span many aspects of care—including identifying risk points in the process of care that require improvements.

A BRIEF HISTORY OF QUALITY

When the ancient Greek physician Hippocrates declared, "First, do no harm!" in the fifth century B.C.E. (Before the Common Era), he was admonishing his peers not to do any intervention that could hurt patients. This seems an obvious and therefore unnecessary directive. Yet even today, doctors and other professionals can easily cause harm. If they don't know what is causing an illness, if they are not aware of certain physical conditions of their patients, if they are wrong in their diagnoses or their cures, if their information is incomplete, if their interventions are not useful, they do harm. Hippocrates was saying that it was the job of the physician to manage, as we would say today, the quality of care given to the patient. Ancient doctors can be said to be the first quality managers.

Fast-forward to the middle of the nineteenth century, when hospitals were doing a brisk and often bad business in managing the safety and quality of care their patients were receiving. Florence Nightingale, during her experience as a nurse in the Crimean War and subsequently, was among the first health care providers to put two and two together and have it add up correctly to four. The 1800s, in England, was an age of science and rational thought (the Age of Reason, it was called), and saw the birth of statistics. People began collecting data and analyzing information, asking why things happen in certain ways and not others.

Connecting the Dots

Florence Nightingale began to make associations. She observed that a soldier had a greater likelihood of dying in a hospital than on the battlefield. Nightingale sought to analyze why this should be, and discovered that sanitary conditions were appalling, ventilation was terrible, cleanliness was disregarded, and so infection spread like wildfire through the buildings. She collected facts, aggregated them, and made causal connections between them. Her analyses were data-driven, based on statistics and evidence.

Doctors who didn't wash their hands as they moved from patient to patient had a greater infection rate and higher rate of mortality than doctors who did. Cause led to effect. Today, all this seems perfectly clear, but the notion of connecting facts, or data elements, with outcomes like mortality was new. With these insights, managing quality became more than the individual physician's responsibility; quality care was shown to be related to the kinds of processes and procedures that permeated the entire health care organization.

Using data to connect the dots between disparate elements (hand washing and mortality, for instance) drove policy and procedures to change, and data were used to assess whether or not the changes made were effective. Nightingale's innovations, not only of care but of analyses of that care, gave rise to the modern notion of quality management. Quality management involves collecting information to assess the quality of care in health care institutions.

Taking Responsibility

The next landmark for quality management occurred in the beginning of the twentieth century, when Dr. Ernest A. Codman suggested that hospitals should be responsible not only for preventing harm but for successful treatment. He said that every patient should be followed in order to determine if the care received had been successful. If it had not been successful, it was the responsibility of the hospital to discover why not, to determine what had gone wrong so that similar failures could be prevented in the future. Codman held the physician and the institution accountable for their actions.

For Codman and his followers, quality was defined by the results of the care delivered, that is, by outcomes. This definition of quality is forward-looking, both in time and conception, requiring institutions (rather than physicians) to be responsible for quality care, and tracking patients after treatment to assess the totality of their care. In addition to this new theoretical model of quality, Codman (who was detested by his peers) developed a methodology for managing the quality of care by using statistical measurements to analyze outcomes.

Outcomes analyses became the basis for defining quality, expanding the idea of quality care from a discussion of process alone to include that of end results. As another quality theoretician, Avedias Donabedian, summed up: quality is determined by the environment of care, the process by which care is delivered, and the outcomes of the interventions.

But whose definition should be used to define a "good" outcome? The physician, who might be looking for a reduction in tumor size or pleased by a particular lab result, or the patient, who wants to feel better, go home, and return to work? If the tumor is reduced but complications from the treatment prevent the patient from returning to normal life, is that a good outcome? Probably not for the patient. If a physician makes a mistake and injures a patient in the course of treatment, that seems easily defined as a poor outcome. But if the physician communicates the misadventure to the patient openly and honestly, and the patient feels fully informed and sympathetic to the physician, and follow-up care successfully heals the patient (a good outcome), the patient may not take legal action (a good outcome for the institution and the physician) and may feel that the physician is trustworthy (a good outcome). Many variables from many sources, both clinical and patient-centered, must be included in the definition of a good outcome.

Outcome and Income

The recent trend to publish hospital report cards has forced health care institutions to collect data about outcomes and make the results available to the public. Imagine that the hospital you work in is not cleaned adequately; the garbage is not removed, or the floors, walls, bathrooms are not washed down adequately. Everyone responsible is aware of this problem, but they wring their hands and say there is not enough money in the budget to hire the staff to do it right.

When a prestigious newspaper such as the *New York Times* reports that the infection rate in this hospital is higher than the state average, and that patients are dying from infection, the report of that outcome drives patients away. Fewer patients mean reduced income for the hospital. Suddenly, money can be found in the budget for cleanliness, because the clinical implications, in this case, infection, have been highlighted for administrators. However, once a hospital or health care organization loses its good name, it is very difficult to recoup. It's a buyer's market out there; therefore the relationship between outcome and income should be recognized.

Infection is a poor outcome, one that involves the activities of many departments—Nursing, Infection Control, Environmental Safety, and others. It is imperative to good management to recognize the connection between the services you provide—or don't provide—and the outcomes to patients. Leadership has the responsibility of providing quality care within a budget. The budget can set limits on what the organization can offer to patients, but not on the quality of the care that is offered.

Administrators and managers need to do a kind of ongoing market analysis in order to understand who is in the population being served and why. Why do patients with certain conditions, for example, cancer or high-risk pregnancies, come to certain hospitals and not to others? Or why is one hospital attracting patients who require high-tech services and another is not? If you ask yourself what is attracting patients and what is driving them elsewhere, you can explore the idea of increasing market share. Quality care attracts patients. It is good business. And every manager's success is judged by results. If you manage a unit that is successful, it is because you have understood your market and are committed to the delivery of quality care for your patients.

Quality Control

In the mid-twentieth century, industry began to delve into quality control issues. The idea was that a manager could control the quality of production or services by controlling the number of mistakes or errors. Focusing on mistakes offers a slightly different perspective on quality than focusing solely on successful outcomes. A manager could measure success by measuring errors; fewer errors equaled a higher-quality product. The goal of the management was to monitor and improve quality (reduce errors) so that costs would be reduced, customers would be satisfied, and products would be standardized and thus manufactured without flaws.

Think about car tires and the way they are manufactured. One factory turns out a high volume of perfect tires, produced without flaws; a second factory has poor management and inadequate processes, and so produces tires that are not up to standard. The outcome might be that the tires manufactured in the second factory have to be recalled because people are getting in accidents and even dying due to faulty tires. Factory one manufactured a quality product; factory two did not.

Even worse would be if the tire company knew that the tires were flawed but because of economics was reluctant to disturb production to investigate the reason for the problem. Disrupting production would certainly have a huge financial impact on the company, but allowing the problem to continue would have a greater one. There would be lawsuits; the government could start monitoring the company, or the company could go bankrupt.

How do you avoid errors in production? It was thought that developing specific standards for high quality and having a methodology to ensure that the standards were met would reduce unwanted variation from the standard. The philosophy was to do it the right way all the time. The focus for quality shifted to standards and variation from standards. Eliminating variation would result in good quality.

It follows that a methodology had to be developed that would measure and monitor the quality of the goods or services produced. In the 1920s, Walter A. Shewhart and W. Edwards Deming developed a model for assessing and improving quality, the Plan-Do-Check-Act (PDCA) model, still used today in health care as a method to develop plans for improvement, implement them, then evaluate them.

Shewhart made use of control charts for determining the success of the improvement efforts. (More about the PDCA and control charts in Chapter Five.) Other scientists (Joseph Juran, Phillip Crosby), working to rebuild Japan's economy after World War II, developed different tools for measuring and monitoring quality. Even today, we use models from the business world, such as Six Sigma, and adapt these models to health care.

MANAGING QUALITY TODAY

But there are important differences between quality in industry and in health care. A patient is not a manufactured widget that can be forced to conform to uniform expectations like an assembly-line product. Nor is the production of good health the same as flying a plane successfully, although comparisons are often made between health care and aviation. Pilots, like doctors, are responsible for human lives, and their skill, training, processes, and equipment all affect the outcome of the flight.

To avoid tragic accidents, the aviation industry took the concept of quality most seriously and developed policies and procedures for preventive maintenance so that the planes were continually checked for proper upkeep. Built-in redundancy was incorporated into monitoring the equipment, so that more than one person confirmed that the plane was perfectly prepared for each flight. Sleep schedules, off times, and alcoholic intake were all supervised so that pilots would be maximally efficient also.

Of course, equipment maintenance, a safe environment, and competency of professional staff are all important aspects of delivering a quality service. However, a patient is not a flight path. A patient is complicated, with a unique physical history and condition. Treatment needs to be tailored to the specific needs of the specific patient. Moreover, the "product" to be delivered to this unique patient is a good outcome. Health care is unusual in that it is the interaction between the patient and the care provided, the consumer and the service, which results in positive outcomes. In the case of aviation, the pilot and crew interact with the machine and the specialist, like the air traffic controller, rather than with the passengers.

When patients participate in their care, outcomes are better than when patients are uninformed or uneducated. If they understand the need to get up and move around after surgery, for example, the outcome is better than if they remain bedridden. If they are unable to follow their discharge instructions because they were poorly informed about the importance of complying with their doctor's directions, they may have to be readmitted to the hospital—a poor outcome. Providing quality in health care is not the same as in manufacturing, industry, or aviation.

Setting Standards

In the beginning of the twentieth century, the American College of Surgeons (ACS) began to publish minimum standards for physicians and initiated a voluntary accreditation program for hospitals. This was the start of external regulatory agencies' monitoring competence and quality of care. In the 1950s the JCAHO (extending the ACS program) published the first standards for hospital accreditation. It is crucial for hospitals to be accredited if they want to receive Medicare reimbursement. Although accreditation is entirely voluntary and optional, few institutions could stay in business without it. Therefore, these standards, which specifically and elaborately define quality, must be met.

The JCAHO standards attempted to normalize the unbalanced relationship between the physician and the hospital. Traditionally, physicians had a free hand in the delivery of care because their economic input into the hospital was vital. If they did not bring in their patients, the hospital would suffer financially. Therefore, physicians were accountable only to themselves and their patients, not to the organization where they practiced medicine. The JCAHO standards forced physicians to be responsible for the quality of care delivered by the hospital with which they were associated. Physicians were expected to participate in hospital activities such as medical staff meetings and to review important areas of practice, such as infection control, medical records, and credentialing, and to participate in mortality and morbidity case conferences.

As JCAHO standards moved beyond monitoring the delivery of quality care to a more problem-oriented approach to care, the agency directed hospitals to collect data to identify *potential* problem areas and to develop corrective actions. The assumption underlying this mandate was that with such a complex organization, problems are inevitable, and anticipating them and providing risk-reduction strategies *in advance* would work to improve outcomes—and thus quality. Today the JCAHO standards encourage organizations to improve the quality of care delivered to patients and improve organizational performance with an emphasis on leadership commitment to quality management data, and with the use of quality measurements and methodologies that can be used to implement improvements and enhance patient safety.

Yet with all the theory and standards regarding the delivery of quality care, it remains somewhat elusive. Health care cannot be said to be exemplary. Just a few years ago, in 1999, the Institute of Medicine published an indictment of the health care industry, suggesting that more than ninety-eight thousand people a year die of medical mistakes in this country. The magnitude of such errors reveals the existence of poor processes that lead inevitably to poor outcomes. Promoting safer practices has provoked private industry and government agencies, such as the Leapfrog Group and the Centers for Medicare and Medicaid Services (CMS), to monitor the delivery of services for successful outcomes. Figure 2.1 highlights the landmarks in the development of quality management theory through the ages, as it increases in complexity and accountability.

Quality Thinking

For years the health care industry has been making use of quality management models and tools to improve the quality of its services. We have seen many trends and theories (quality improvement, quality assurance, total quality management, continuous quality improvement) about the way to collect data, interpret performance, and plan for improvement. But providing quality care involves more than data measurement and interpretation, and more than monitoring compliance with regulations. Working within a quality management model, health care managers are expected to champion improvement efforts and improve processes, using the PDCA methodology.

How can quality be managed so that the delivery of care is excellent? These past decades prove that knowing the tools and techniques of quality management does not automatically ensure the delivery of quality care. Understanding quality involves thinking about care in an objective way, always keeping in mind that the end product should be good outcomes for all patients. Often, improvement requires changing behaviors, including entrenched behaviors of thought. Managers, along with their staff, need to embrace new ideas, to "think outside the box," to encourage and empower critical thinking and discourage worn-out, rote responses. The PDCA cycle is so productive because it makes room for new learning about the delivery of care while changing performance.

There is no quick fix for care that needs improvement. Learning is a slow process, occurring over time and involving intellectual activity and new practices. Think of what is involved in learning to ride a bike or make an omelet: principles have to be understood and then practiced; competence comes with repeated, sometimes unsuccessful trials. Managing quality involves a kind of team learning so that change can occur without ignoring the complexity of the services that have to be delivered.

Quality, then, can be thought of as a culture or mindset, one that involves a kind of intellectual openness to problem solving and improving

Hippocrates	Florence Nightingale	Ernest A. Codman	Walter A. Shewhart
500 B.C.E.	Mid-1850s	1914	1920s
Do No Harm	• Data • Cause-Effect	• Treatment Should Be Successful	• Plan • Do • Check • Act

Joint Commission (JCAHO)	W. Edwards Deming and Joseph Juran	Avedis Donabedian and Phillip Crosby	JCAHO
1950	1960	1970	1980
Standards for Hospital Accreditation	• Statistical Models • Total Quality Management • Plan, Control, and Improve • Standards Lead to Improved Quality	• Structure • Process • Outcome • Zero Defects	• Potential Problems • Corrective Action

Institute of Medicine	Private Industry	Centers for Medicare and Medicaid Services
1990	2000	2003
• Building Safer Systems • Improving Chronic Conditions • Educate Public About Errors	• Leapfrog • Business Recommend Safety Goals and Practices	• Consumer Choice • Public Reporting • Hospital Report Cards • Pay for Quality

Figure 2.1.   Landmarks in Defining Quality Management.

processes. Working within such a culture, along with the quality tools and techniques and in concert with the regulatory requirements, managers can deliver the care and services they are charged to deliver across a broad range of situations and conditions. Satisfying the physician (clinical performance), the patient (quality of life, outcomes), and the health system leadership (accreditation, efficiency, costs), a quality approach becomes a dynamic and robust methodology that managers can use to empower their staff to think creatively and critically.

Quality Data

The question remains, however, How can you *prove* that you are delivering good care and responding to the different expectations of the physicians you work with, the patients you serve, your own manager, and other departments within the organization? The answer involves the objectivity of data. Data don't play politics or respond to social pressures. If you establish standards rooted in science, collect information regarding services, and compare the standards that you developed through a team approach to others, you then have a framework that can inarguably define the quality of your product. Science, both in establishing guidelines and in statistical analysis, anchors quality care.

It is very difficult to remain unmoved by social and political pressures in a high-stress working environment like health care. It is only natural to try to please your boss and perhaps not rock any boats. If you focus on the quality of care delivered, no doubt someone will be displeased, because quality, especially the framework we are putting forth here, requires new modes of thought, which might lead you to step on some toes. However, quality data are entirely objective because facts tell the truth.

A quality framework creates accountability for performance and sets expectations for staff. The great value of this approach to quality is that it can be used to change behavior and to implement new processes and procedures. It promotes a way of looking at a problem that goes around political and social concerns and interpersonal dynamics. Working with a clear objective—to deliver excellent care and service—you can define success as well as failure.

As a manager, you don't want to accept the status quo as the best you can do; you want to improve—you want to be excellent. Your data, then, are collected not for compliance (for example, lab data) but for change and improvement. You can measure a process because it is broken or inefficient, or you can measure processes because you want to improve them. We believe that data and measurements should be collected in a principled way (based on the PDCA model) in order to institute changes.

Quality Assessment

Whatever type of service or unit you manage, your role as a manager is to deliver good outcomes, maintain a pleasant environment, provide processes for crisis reduction, ensure the proper utilization of resources, and meet the discharge disposition of your patients in a timely way, while maintaining a high level of quality care. If you manage an oncology service or unit, for example, how can you ascertain if you are doing as well as you should, or if you could do better? First you need to collect information to understand and analyze what the care is like on your unit.

Who are your patients? What are their diagnoses? What are the typical comorbidities common to this patient population? What services are required for care? What problems have arisen? How were they handled? What is the competency level of your staff? Are resources being used appropriately?

Once you collect this information, you still may not be able to evaluate if the care you are delivering is excellent or not. If you know that a certain percentage of your patients has pain management problems, how do you know if that is a reasonable or acceptable outcome? You might want to compare your data to the data regarding care in other similar units. You might want to look at such readily available data as length of stay or patient satisfaction to see if your data compare well to nationally established standards, often called *benchmarks*. The other question you might ask is if you need to get involved in clinical matters. The answer is yes, but not at the individual patient level. You need to address the global issues that can make your patients satisfied with the care your service provides.

Asking Quality Questions

The managers' role is to ask "why" and "why not" in search of ways to improve the services they deliver and to meet the goals established in the organization's strategic plan. If your inquiries reveal that your oncology patients experience terrible fatigue and nausea with chemotherapy treatments, how might you improve their situation? As a manager, you always want to improve.

But before you can make improvements, you need facts, and that means you ask more questions. Is it normal to be fatigued? Is it acceptable? Is fatigue experienced by all chemo patients, or is it as a result of certain treatments and not others? What can be done to relieve it? Are the current processes adequate? Are the staff and environment responsive? Is the fatigue causing any problems on the unit? Is the staff/patient ratio reasonable to handle the consequences of this problem?

You are not expected to know all the answers to all the questions you ask, but as a manager, you are expected to develop resources as needed. You can form a multidisciplinary team of experts to discuss the issues and assign staff to research the literature on fatigue and oncology patients. Once the current practice is delineated and the issues that warrant improvement identified, you can begin to plan for change. Perhaps if nausea is an expected and inevitable result of treatment, then new protocols should be developed to care for patients who are experiencing this problem. If palliative care measures need to be developed so that your patients are more comfortable, what would they consist of?

The information your team has collected enables you to make informed decisions about staffing ratios, bed utilization, ancillary services, education of patients, families, and staff, medication needs, nutritional involvement, or alternative therapies available to manage discomfort. Moreover, you can ask for support and resources in a nonrandom way. You can provide objective evidence that additional services are needed. You can make the case for change.

Don't congratulate yourself, yet. This is not the end of the story. Once you begin to implement new practices, you need to collect data to evaluate their impact on an ongoing basis. Monitoring the effectiveness of new protocols focuses attention on the improvements in the delivery of care. If successful, your changes—the data—can be communicated to other units within the hospital or system.

Another example. You receive a call at 6 A.M. about an incident in the Emergency Department (ED) where a specimen was not delivered in a timely way to the laboratory. You try and collect the facts. Instead of keeping the specimen in the refrigerator until the next routine pickup, staff wrapped the specimen in a towel and left it on a desk. Why? Upon investigation you discover that a physician was leaning against the refrigerator talking to the patient's family, and the nurse did not want to interrupt or intrude. The towel was to prevent visitors from seeing the specimen. The delay caused the patient to have another (unnecessary) biopsy—the improper storage meant that the specimen could not be used for diagnosis.

You call Quality Management and Risk Management to report the incident. But this is your unit, and so this is your problem. What do you, as the manager, do? You can fire the nurse who forgot to deliver the specimen on time, or you can expose her to the blame and shame response of her colleagues. ("How could you be so stupid and careless?") But no. You are a good manager who works within a quality framework with a team who believes in a quality culture. Therefore you begin to ask pertinent questions. How often does such an error occur? For this particular staff person? Under what circumstances does it occur? A good manager will do a root cause analysis to figure out what had an impact on the problem with the intention of improving the process.

Improvement is intended to change the process or the environment in which a problem, like the misplaced specimen just described, occurred. Removing the individual responsible would not solve the problem or change anything, although such a response might instill fear in your employees that if they make a mistake and admit it, their jobs would be in jeopardy. Real improvement attacks those elements that provided the opportunity for the incident to have occurred. Why did the doctor need to speak with the patient's family near the specimen refrigerator? Should the refrigerator be moved to a less public location? Improvement is difficult and time-consuming and needs to be monitored and measured to see if the changes made are effective.

Getting Quality Responses

Now that your initial questions have been answered, you can begin to get a handle on some of the issues that caused the incident. The next step is to prioritize what to do. If the room was too crowded, a new process flow has to be designed, implemented, and tested for effectiveness. If the nurse was too shy, staff education has to occur, for both physicians and nurses, stressing the importance to the patient of communication and carrying out responsibilities. If the nurse was distracted and asked to do something else and then forgot to return for the specimen, your staff need a procedure for following through assigned tasks, even under fire. Was there not enough staff present to do what needed to be done? Perhaps the rest of the staff relaxed their vigilance because this did not seem like a crisis event. Constant vigilance for details needs to be inculcated into the staff.

Other processes have to be analyzed as well. Is there a way to decrease the number of steps involved in getting a specimen from the

ED to the lab? Is new technology required (or old technology, such as a pneumatic tube)? If so, what data would show time savings and error reduction in the delivery of specimens? Is there a procedure whereby the receiving lab alerts the floor that an expected specimen hasn't arrived? All this information would promote change, creating greater efficiency, utilization, accuracy, and timeliness.

CREATING A CULTURE OF QUALITY

In any working environment informal peer pressure can interfere with management's goals. Quality can mediate between the two. For example, if a member of the staff makes a medication error, there may be informal censure from peers, or even a wall of silence as the staff unites in a cover-up for the manager. If the problem becomes serious enough for an error to reach the patient, a formal structure is mandated, as sentinel events are required to be reported in a particular framework.

A good manager will recognize the difference between formal and informal processes and use quality methods to develop a bridge between the two, perhaps by encouraging a blame-free environment or rewarding staff for identifying small problems before they become serious ones. The attitude of the manager is all-important in eliciting trust and respect from the staff. Shared expectations for excellence and a genuine respect for patient care will help the manager create a culture of quality.

Viewing the Big Picture

With information regarding the environment, technology, equipment, patients, staffing needs, and competency requirements of the staff on the unit, and understanding the expectations of the organization as defined by its mission and vision statements, the manager can develop processes for improving care even in the most difficult situations, such as a busy and crowded Emergency Department. Difficult situations challenge the manager to manage well. The challenge can seem overwhelming, but that is precisely when having deliberate processes in place can be of most value.

Say you have a flow problem. Patients are spending long periods of time in the ED waiting to be seen and treated. Obviously, some process is failing. If you are a clinician, you will find it tempting to step in to help to try and improve the situation. But if a manager does that, becoming a member of the caretaking team, who is left in charge and supervising? Who is in a position to see the big picture? Lack of supervision can create additional problems in an already problem-ridden environment.

Quality management methods can be brought to bear to improve the situation. First, information is necessary. It may seem counterintuitive in a busy and chaotic situation to stop and brainstorm with your team, because delays and associated problems could be further increased. However, until a rational process is developed, based on information about the process that is in place, improvement is impossible.

The patient flow issues must be analyzed with the goal of understanding the bottlenecks in the process that prevent all patients from being evaluated properly and in a timely fashion. The manager and team have to gather information regarding the environment—is the space adequate to accommodate the stream of people coming in? Is it clean? Is the staffing adequate? Information is also necessary about timeliness of care—is there a holdup in triaging patients? Do the appropriate consultations occur in a timely way? Are tests or technology causing a backup? What is the average time a patient waits before being assessed and treated? How long does a patient stay in the ED?

Once information about these and other appropriate variables is collected and analyzed, the manager has to focus on issues surrounding getting patients to their destination. The manager should meet with the floor managers and unit managers to identify potential obstacles to moving patients quickly onto the units. Is Housekeeping bed turnover a problem? Or is the delay in discharging patients? What is having an impact?

If you try and fix the situation patient by patient and problem by problem, every day will bring new patients with new problems. The solution has to be developed on a higher level, that is, on a process level, involving people from many disciplines, from the ED, Radiology, Ancillary Services, Social Work, Housekeeping, and Nursing, to name just a few. Until the big picture is viewed, the bottlenecks will not be easily identified. Data, over a period of time, will reveal where the problems are and thus where improvements can be targeted to the appropriate issues.

The goal in this example is to improve the flow of patients through the ED. What processes can be measured to see if that goal is met? Say you measure time from entry to discharge, and you find that time for each patient is decreasing. Do you pat yourself on the back and assume the problem has been solved? Not so fast. You have to consider the bigger picture and beware of superficial success.

Perhaps the ED is letting patients go prematurely. How could you determine if that were the case? You can collect data about how many patients left without being seen—those patients may not have been counted in your data about time of entry to discharge (since they were not seen, they were not discharged). Or you could collect information about returns to the ED within seventy-two hours. A good manager never rests on assumed laurels. If you keep drilling down, asking why or why not, and collecting data, you will be in a position to develop improved processes that can make an impact on the way all the patients are treated.

Analyzing Processes of Care

Good processes result in good outcomes, and managers are evaluated by the processes they manage. Regardless of whether the unit is busy, or the shift is changing, or everything is calm, or a crisis strikes, a good manager has processes that enable the unit to run smoothly. A manager can't control people and can't control disease, but can and should control the processes involved in the delivery of care. Without good processes, you can expect poor results or even adverse events.

Data will illustrate whether or not you have good processes. For example, if you manage a unit with patients who have community-acquired pneumonia (CAP), what is your goal, your definition of providing quality care? Perhaps it is to reduce fever, improve breathing, and reduce pain. Government guidelines for CAP recommend that antibiotics be given within a certain time span. Is it important to you to meet that evidence-based recommendation? If you can demonstrate, through data, that the CAP patients on your unit have received antibiotics in a timely way, you have a concrete measure of your unit's performance. You can compare your data to the national benchmark, and if your results are better, you have proof that your care is outstanding. Good outcomes are the result of good processes.

However, if your data reveal opportunities for improvement, you need to drill down and start asking pertinent questions. Figure 2.2 shows that in the months of January and February, on a single unit, the number of patients with CAP increased, and there was also a delay in antibiotic administration. In March and April, on the other hand, the benchmark was met. What caused the difference? It is the manager's job to investigate and understand the delivery of care.

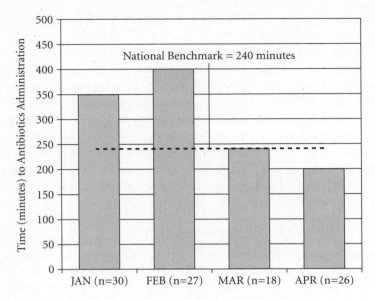

**Figure 2.2.   Community-Acquired Pneumonia:
Antibiotic Timing on a Medical Unit.**

Several possibilities should be explored. Were data on each incident accurate and collected uniformly across the four-month period? Did patients receive the antibiotic in the ED rather than on the unit, so the source of the delay was there? Was the pharmacy involved? Did its method of delivery change in any way? On the unit, was there a change in staff? Was the staff large enough to respond to the higher volume during the higher-volume months? Perhaps as a result of data collection, the problem with antibiotic delivery was revealed and the staff responded. Was there an educational effort between February and March? Collecting data provides the manager with information with which to analyze the processes of care.

Set an Example

Within the past decade, the health care industry has evolved to the point where health care institutions are expected to explicitly define their mission and vision, and to articulate their goals and expectations for delivering quality care. Managers are responsible for embedding these goals into the daily processes of patient care, for setting expectations, and for educating their staff appropriately about how to reach the goals.

Having your own definition of what it means to provide quality care in your department or in the service you deliver promotes accountability and is a prescription for success. Success is the delivery of care that results in good outcomes for the patient. Good outcomes for the patient lead to increased revenue for the organization, because physicians, staff, and patients are attracted to a quality organization.

As your staff sees that you value quality and are committed to developing good processes, you will set a direction for their work that will serve you, them, the patients, and the organization well. There will be less chaos because processes will be in place, and there will be fewer errors because the delivery of care will be carefully monitored and assessed, and when necessary improved. Working within a quality framework makes managing manageable.

SUMMARY

Delivering quality in health care includes taking all of the following steps:

- Comply with regulatory standards.
- Use comparative measures to assess performance.
- Balance the expectations of physicians, patients, and the organization.
- Remember that the patient always comes first.
- Develop processes and measurements that span many aspects of care.
- Use objective information to assess the quality of care delivered.
- Analyze processes and outcomes of care.
- Be responsive to the expectations of the community served.
- Measure variation from standards of care.
- Include the patient in the process of care.
- Anticipate problems and develop corrective action.
- Champion improvement efforts.
- Collaborate with other departments on improvement initiatives.

- Assess and improve care through the PDCA methodology.
- Bridge formal and informal processes involved in the delivery of care.
- Develop good processes that lead to good outcomes.

Things to Think About

- You are the manager of an oncology service, and your manager wants proof that you are doing your job well. What proof would you offer?
- A patient commits suicide on the medical unit you manage. How would you handle the investigation?
- You realize that your staff is not forthcoming about their problems or the patient care issues they discover. How would you improve the situation?

CHAPTER THREE

Information and Prioritization

In Chapter Two we suggested the kinds of questions that managers need to ask to do their jobs effectively within a quality management framework. In this chapter, we turn to ways the manager might productively evaluate and use the answers to those questions.

Managers in health care have no scarcity of information. On the contrary, information and data are available from many sources. There are treatment details in the medical record, nursing data in shift reports, errors documented in incident reports, patient satisfaction survey data revealing people's experience with the delivery of care, complaints and compliments from patients and their families, quality indicators collected to satisfy regulatory requirements, as well as diverse information from external databases.

In New York State, the Statewide Planning and Research Cooperative System (SPARCS) database collects data regarding demographics, diagnoses, discharge disposition, length of stay, and case mix index for patients across the state based on billing data. The state Peer Review Organization (PRO) reports information about specific clinical quality indicators, such as time of aspirin administration for patients with myocardial infarction, and establishes benchmarks for comparable institutions within the region. The Centers for Medicare and Medicaid Services (CMS) provides similar benchmarks nationally and anticipates publicly reporting outcomes for specific diseases and implementing quality measurements in the ambulatory setting (that is, in physician offices). Furthermore, CMS is considering offering financial incentives to organizations that can prove themselves successful in treating these diseases. New York State provides health care organizations with risk-adjusted mortality rates for specific diseases. Other data, internal to the organization, might also be available—from the laboratory, or about equipment, or radiology and pathology reports, information about nutrition requirements and food delivery, social services issues, staffing data, medical test results, and so on.

In fact, so much information is available that a responsible professional could become paralyzed from the sheer volume and speed of the flow. Like the suffering manager in Figure 3.1, you may feel as though you're getting too much information to take it in. In sociology, this phenomenon is referred to as *alienation*. Surrounded by information, you may not be able to focus on a clear direction for your actions and may end up sitting in your office with your door closed, staring at a wall. This unproductive behavior is common in chaotic and seemingly uncontrollable situations.

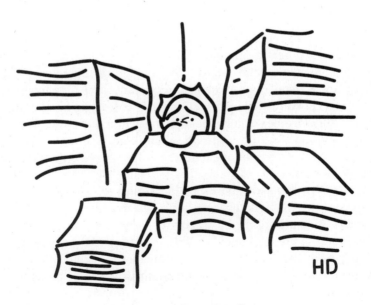

Figure 3.1.   Data Overflow.

To avoid information overload, it is most important that you provide yourself with tools to help you control the wealth of information coming at you and to evaluate what you need to address. You want a principled method to determine what data will be most productive for you and how to best use the information you collect. You need a tool designed to help you filter and prioritize information.

To return to the overcrowded Emergency Department example, say you (as the manager) turn to the Quality Management Department in distress because you have been receiving repeated deficiencies from the state DOH, despite having developed corrective actions and despite ongoing monitoring. What should you do? Several immediate responses are possible in a case like this. Someone might think you were simply incapable and incompetent and should not be in such an important managerial position. Or perhaps the state inspectors were unreasonable to expect miracles in such crowded conditions, with inadequate staffing and too few beds available to address the needs of the increasing number of patients. It is always easy to cast blame.

Both types of response are unhelpful to you and to the patients in the ED. A more reasoned response is to question the forces that contribute to the overcrowding and to gather data for analysis about gatekeeping. Who evaluates patients for ED services, and what criteria are used for admission? When there is a sudden avalanche of patients, what process is in place to maintain control? Is admission on a first-come, first-served basis or on a specific set of clinical indicators? Is the person responsible for triage well trained? Who is accountable if patients leave before being evaluated, or are seen, discharged, and then readmitted to the hospital? Since your ED service is interrelated with others, you should be examining processes of care in such areas as the Intensive Care Units (ICUs), telemetry, the operating rooms, and on the floors. Delays or inefficiencies in any one of these areas could contribute to problems occurring in the ED.

ESTABLISHING CRITERIA

Once you gather information, what do you do with it? In other words, how do you assess the value of the information you receive and then use the information to make intelligent decisions about improving performance? Information closely related to your clearly defined and reasonable goals and to your priorities will be most important to you.

Think about buying a car and choosing from among the many available models which car would be best for you. One of the reasons the automakers offer so many options is that different people desire different qualities in a car, depending on what is important to them and what their goals are. If your primary concern is to have a superb safety record, you might concentrate on that, but if your goal is to find the vehicle with the most bells and whistles, or the one that can accommodate a family of six with two large dogs and the need to use a VCR on the road, or the most economical one to run in terms of gas mileage, you look for that.

Once you define your goals, you need to collect information that will have an impact on your decision. Information can be gathered from various sources. Some people go directly to *Consumer Reports* for data regarding safety records, gas mileage statistics, weight, price, and the availability of personal comfort devices like lumbar supports. Others talk to their friends and amass information that is entirely different, related to the stereo system, the speed capacity, the tire size, and the appearance.

One set of criteria is not objectively more valuable or useful than the other, nor is one source of information obviously superior. The value of the information and its source is determined by the customer's goals and requirements. If you are selling cars, you need to know who your customers are, what their expectations are, and what criteria you should use to meet those expectations. If you are managing a health care unit or delivering a health care service, you also need to know who your customers are and what are their expectations or goals.

If you're having the sort of problems described in the ED example, you are failing to meet your customers' expectations. Most patients who come to a hospital ED are sick, and it is the manager's job to address this fact. The goal of the ED patient is to be treated quickly and to feel better as a result of that treatment. If people leave the ED without being able to return to their lives or perform their jobs, they have not been well served.

Know Your Customers

Regardless of what department or service you manage, the patient is always your primary customer. Therefore, any information that might result in better care and a shorter hospitalization for each patient is crucial to meeting expectations. In addition to the patient, the institution is also your customer, in a sense, because it is the manager's responsibility to promote the institution's goals and ensure that they are reached. In a quality hospital, mission and vision statements are not just fancy rhetoric, they actually define the relationship between the organization and the patients. Such a definition can provide valuable direction for how to establish priorities for your department or service and thus inform you about the type of information you need if you are to reach these goals.

If, for example, your leadership is committed to a "zero defect" policy regarding the delivery of service, you might put your energy and resources into increasing efficiency, productivity, and quality. If the mission of your organization is to increase patient satisfaction (what is called "service quality"), you might want to introduce patient-friendly services such as patient advocates, patient education videos, and so on. Today, most hospitals attempt to satisfy both goals because of the expectations of the government, employers, and consumers who use report cards of clinical and service quality indicators to make choices about where to go for health care services.

The institution may well expect managers to collect and analyze information that promotes its articulated goals, especially information that helps the administrative leadership allocate resources appropriately. Without data, it is difficult to know how to prioritize expenditures. At a recent Finance Committee meeting at the NS-LIJHS, the discussion focused on the financial benefits of reducing length of stay (LOS). Data revealed that there had been no reduction over a period of time, even though the administration had invested money and resources to change processes and improve roles and function to enable a better throughput from the ED to the floor to discharge. The Board, understandably, was dissatisfied with the lack of return on their investment.

This occasion presented the managers with an opportunity for accountability. You can attempt to justify the lack of change in LOS by saying that care is complex and difficult to measure—and be regarded with skepticism by the members of the Board—or you can provide analytic information that explains the situation. In today's health care market, the demand for information that accounts for the relationship between cost and care is increasing. A good manager gathers information that addresses this relationship.

At the organizational level, as well as at the patient level, providing information that the hospital is doing everything possible to prevent incidents may also be required from the manager. Positive and negative publicity is usually based on such data.

Quality information that is required for compliance with state and federal regulations is also expected. Your own manager or supervisor may demand information proving that you are running your department well, keeping within the budget, delivering appropriate care, and educating staff. The Quality Management Department may require certain information and analysis about performance, processes, incidents, or events. In sum, a manager may be required to manage (that is, collect and analyze) information that responds to the needs of the organization, and that helps improve care for patients, is responsive to costs, enables problems to be anticipated, and establishes best practices for the delivery of service. That's a great deal of information to manage!

Sharing Information

Gathering and analyzing information is not enough. For information to be useful it needs to be communicated—up, down, and sideways, and related to specific goals and objectives. Managers have to relay information to their own managers, to other care providers, and to support staff. Information, depending on its nature, goes to the medical boards, the administration, and external agencies. The information that needs to be transmitted must be objective and quantifiable, and must explain clinical phenomena and promote accountability.

In the ED example, if you'd had data to bring to administrative leadership about patients who left without being evaluated because of lengthy wait times, or data that showed that patients were returning within seventy-two hours—indicating they were being sent away prematurely—that would have allowed you to make a more convincing case for resources and improvement efforts than just repeating that the ED is overcrowded and that everyone is doing the best they can. With demographic and clinical data regarding who comes to the ED with what kinds of problems and when, and who leaves before being admitted, and why, and which member of the health care team saw the would-be patients and what triage level were they identified at, all collected over time (at least a month), a manager can make educated assumptions about the processes that are making an impact in the delivery of services and possible interventions for improvements, and can then propose concrete improvements to administration.

In our large, multihospital health care system, managers from units within each hospital report quality care priorities to their managers, who report to the hospital quality director, who in turn meets with quality directors from other hospitals across the system to determine goals and priorities. System committees made up of administrators, medical leadership, nurses, quality management staff, and trustees meet to discuss quality reports from all the hospitals. This committee structure moves information effectively from the caregiver at the bedside to the Board of Trustees. All this information informs decision making at all levels from the individual unit to the health care system, and is used to identify problems, formulate programs for improvement, and change policies and procedures. This is as it should be; information needs to be translated into action.

MAKING IMPROVEMENTS

Data, left unanalyzed, are not very informative about anything. Data need to be related to outcomes and to accountability. Without data, it is very difficult to change behaviors or to ensure that patient care is improved. Sometimes crises (financial or clinical) can force change, but if such change is accomplished without regard to quality data, patient care might suffer.

Data collection is required to support supervision of the delivery of care, ensure consistency, and monitor results. Collecting data for regulatory reasons is different from ensuring that proper care is delivered (although the two might lead to similar results). Quality data are used for assessing performance and to identify opportunities for improvement, with the assumption that in the delivery of your scope of care, you meet the expectations of your patient population, their families, and the community. Again, this requires the gathering and analysis of a great deal of information.

Therefore it behooves managers to learn how to identify, collect, and interpret data in order to make the information they communicate useful. Data analysis is vital for identifying areas to target for improvement, for evaluating performance improvement efforts, for understanding adverse outcomes (for example, determining if an event was isolated or part of a trend), and for evaluating the scope of care.

Juggling Competing Agendas

An example from our system about how data help us prioritize improvement programs involves the ICUs. Administration had the impression (with no hard data, one has only impressions) that the ICUs, which require vast financial, technical, and human resources, were not being appropriately utilized. Expenses were increasing, as was LOS. Quality Management was asked to collaborate with the ICU managers and supervisors to evaluate the situation and to determine if improvements in utilization and resource consumption could be made. Until information could be acquired, we had no basis on which to make recommendations.

Administrative data were not sufficiently sensitive or finely grained to detail the causes of the rising expense and to gauge if it was appropriate. Quality Management staff began biweekly rounds to directly observe the situation in the ICUs. Often direct observation, what is called in the social sciences *participant observation,* is the best methodology to use to evaluate a situation. We saw patients sitting up in bed and reading newspapers, and questioned why such individuals required the complex and costly service of an ICU.

Identifying an issue for correction or improvement is difficult enough, but persuading the administration to support an effort to change physician practices can be even more challenging. Administration was reluctant to interfere with physician practice, since ICU admission was a medical responsibility, and physicians did not appreciate being second-guessed regarding their patient admission decisions. Although the ICU managers and the Quality Management staff believed that the ICU was being used inappropriately, they needed strong arguments to overcome ingrained beliefs and practices.

Administrative and medical leadership had to be convinced first of all that a problem existed and then that a deliberate process to admit and discharge patients and improve patient flow was needed to address the problem. Further, the medical and nursing staff at the bedside had to be persuaded that a change in practice was necessary—that not all patients, regardless of acuity of illness, should be admitted to the ICU. We needed data to evaluate the severity of illness and the appropriateness of care. Changing practice can result in disorganization on the unit, supplying another challenge for the manager. Established routines help caregivers cope with the pressures involved in the delivery of care, and even improvements disrupt routines.

Using Data to Drive Improvement

We found that physicians were admitting patients to the ICU, not according to any established admission criteria, but simply because it had open beds, a 1:2 nursing ratio, and technology that translated into better care from the physician's point of view than what was generally available on a medical or surgical floor. How would a manager be in a position to override a physician's decision, especially since physician admissions are crucial to the hospital's financial survival? A powerful weapon for a determined manager in this situation is the objectivity of data.

Learning how to use comparative data as an effective tool to influence physician behavior can give the manager enough leverage to promote change. Professional staff, when confronted with objective information that makes sense to them, generally react positively. But this process can also meet with resistance because such use of data contradicts the notion that medicine is an art based on subjective experience, and therefore not amenable to objective measurement. Rather than using data to promote collective accountability, many physicians prefer a kind of individual accountability, revealed through malpractice claims or peer review, to deal with problems in the delivery of care.

However, regulatory requirements and the use of quality management methodology can override administrative and physician reluctance to change practices, because the JCAHO and other regulatory agencies require data to monitor performance and provide a framework for improvement efforts. Data must be aggregated and analyzed on an ongoing basis, and the organization is expected to compare its performance with other sources of information. Therefore, the manager and the Quality Management Department can become partners in assessing and improving care on a unit.

In addition, it is expected that a multidisciplinary team including physicians and nurses will collect the required data and illustrate improvement efforts. Participation in data collection and analysis has the further advantage of increasing the investment, what is termed the *buy in,* of the professional staff. Data must be appropriate to address the defined goals. In the ICU example, the goal was to ensure proper utilization of services. To accomplish this, we needed to formulate admission and discharge criteria, and to compare the services delivered in our ICUs with those of other ICUs across the nation.

Assessing Present Practices

After researching the options, a multidisciplinary team recommended that a data management system called APACHE (an acronym for Acute, Physiology, Age, Chronic Health Evaluation) be used to provide objective and consistent information regarding care in the ICUs. The Quality Management leadership argued for its effectiveness in providing information that would improve resource utilization and reduce costs to the institution, and convinced the CEO that return on the investment would be high in terms of decreased length of stay, more appropriate use of beds, and improved flow of patients from the ICU to the floor units.

The APACHE system enabled caregivers to collect invaluable descriptive and clinical information concerning patient demographics, severity of illness, appropriate levels of care, and patient outcomes. These data could then be compared to other hospitals and hospital systems throughout the nation.

The managers' role in evaluating ICU care was critical, from planning for the implementation of this new database to training the staff on how to use it. Staff time and responsibilities required reallocation to incorporate the APACHE system into the daily routine of the unit. The new technology could not be put in place without managerial support since information brings new ideas about care that changes normal or usual practice.

Sociology recognizes that an organization will have a formal structure (as shown in the organization chart) in which roles and responsibilities are prescribed by Human Resources, and a more informal structure based on interaction among staff. The success of a new practice depends on the informal organization and on staff allegiance to their manager. To make change and implement improved practices, the manager had to enlist the support of the ICU staff so that everyone understood the value of data collection and was willing to participate in the improvement effort, which was time-consuming and which provided benefits that were not immediately realized.

Quality Management staff worked with the managers and the ICU staff to educate them about data collection techniques, the use of uniform definitions and calculations, and—most important—on how to utilize tools for the analysis and interpretation of the collected data.

Improving Practices

The data provided objective information about resource utilization in the ICUs and revealed the need for establishing stringent admission and discharge criteria. Physicians could not simply use the ICU for monitoring their patients. According to the regulatory agencies, patients had to meet certain clinical criteria to be admitted to an ICU. The data on severity of illness scaled according to an index, coupled with the comparison of hospital data to the national database, had a profound effect on changing physician behavior so that admissions were reduced and staff used more effectively.

Data helped convince physicians that their patients could be treated in other units in the hospital. Nurse educators shifted their focus toward such issues as establishing weaning protocols for patients on ventilators and training staff in the new protocols. Quality of care improved while costs decreased and resources were more appropriately allocated. Data accomplish this: they mediate among cost, quality, and resources. Most important, data influence the opinions and practices of the professional staff while providing managers with a yardstick for measuring the performance of their service. With data in hand, managers could illustrate that the care being delivered in their ICUs was appropriate and that patients were being treated effectively. When improvements were instituted, the data helped assess their impact.

Any data collected and analyzed for improvement should be focused on a goal, should shed light on the problems in your department, and develop potential areas for improvement. With objective information, you can drill down to assess where you want your resources (both financial and personnel) and improvement efforts to be. The improvements that were made in ICU utilization—new admission and discharge criteria, step-down units, improved nursing education, standardized ventilator-weaning protocols—were based on facts rather than on impressions.

MAKING CHOICES

Obviously, not all information is equal in importance. Some types may be more meaningful at certain times than others, or more critical for successful patient outcomes, or have a higher priority than others for clinical or administrative reasons. As we have said, your specific goals direct your improvement efforts, and your improvement efforts indicate the data you should collect and analyze. You need to balance your immediate and critical priorities with longer-term priorities, all the while dealing with the information that is relevant to the daily functioning of your unit or service.

If you note an incident, perhaps a medical error that had no sequelae (adverse consequences) to the patient but served as a warning to alert you that some process or procedure was vulnerable to error and required improvement or staff member education, you need to gather information immediately in order to best manage the crisis situation. You want to know how this incident occurred. If medication was involved, you want to determine if it was a process problem related to the Pharmacy, a nursing administration error, a prescription error, a transcription error, or something else. Until you can establish the reason for the error, you can't provide a solution.

If the error was rooted in the Pharmacy, you can alert Pharmacy staff that a particular medication was involved in an incident and develop a procedure so that future incidents can be avoided. For example, a medication could be moved to a special "red flagged" section, or could require special cross-checks and confirmations. During a crisis, you deal with the crisis, putting out the fire. Your goal is to gather information to identify the root cause of the problem without interrupting the normal work flow of your unit.

Other problems may come to your attention through complaints, or through incident reports in the professional literature, or you may define opportunities for improvement from your own observation. If you become aware of flaws within your scope of service, you need to prioritize an improvement initiative on a long-term basis. You may need to revisit your policies and redefine your department's objectives; you may need to introduce supervision and education for employees or delineate new lines of accountability. These long-term policies have to take into account budgetary restrictions and Human Resources requirements.

In the Pharmacy incident example, on a longer-term basis and depending on budget restrictions, you might want to encourage computerized physician order entry tools be purchased and then develop an education program to train physicians and other personnel to use these tools to the best advantage of the patient and the organization. Although this is not a quick fix for your medication error—it may take many years to implement—it might be an important future priority. Alternatively, introducing new technology or processes may create unanticipated problems, which is why you always need to evaluate the improvement to make sure you are achieving the desired goal.

Evaluating Improvement Priorities

To make the best use of information for short-term or long-term improvements, it is useful to establish some standards that help you prioritize the relative value of your data. Prioritization is not a simple task because the complexity and interrelationship of services delivered in health care often make it difficult to determine what criteria to use to meet the many expectations of your multiple customers. You don't want to implement cost reduction procedures if they may result in risks to patient safety. As a manager, you always have to balance among personnel, budget, risk, satisfaction, clinical outcomes, events, and goals. Therefore, you need to define a set of criteria to determine if the information related to a particular process or function is of high or low priority for improvement.

To make the task more sensible, the JCAHO has suggested prioritization criteria for objectifying potential problems, indicating that since most organizations have limited resources, managers must make choices about which data to collect and what processes to monitor. The JCAHO recommends that improvement initiatives and associated data collection efforts focus on processes that are *high-risk,* such as those addressing heart attacks, *high-volume,* such as congestive heart failure, or *problem-prone,* such as treating chronic diseases like diabetes that involve several specialists.

Organizing information for prioritization requires thoughtful planning. Start by assessing your processes along the suggested lines. What is high risk or high volume in your scope of care? For example, imagine that you manage a medical or surgical unit in a hospital and patient satisfaction surveys have alerted you that patients are unhappy with the timing of food delivery. As a manager, you want to evaluate whether or not this issue should be a priority for your performance improvement efforts. But to understand the scope of the problem, you need to gather more information. You might want to determine whether or not your patients' health is at risk if their food is not delivered in a timely way; in other words, is food delivery a safety and health issue or a social comfort issue?

Perhaps some of your patients suffer from diabetes or other diseases that interact with food, or they require medication that is associated—or not associated—with food intake (for example, on an empty stomach, with milk). Once you understand what outcomes result from delayed food delivery, you need to explore the underlying causes, the *why's.* Since food is not being delivered on time, you want to know why not, and investigate if this is a staffing problem, an equipment problem, a competency issue, or a process problem. Will more staff be required? Or different technology? Will improving the process involve a great deal of money or simply involve better education for the staff? You need to acquire data.

Information about your patients' diabetes might help you determine whether food delivery is a high priority. The more specific the information, the more detailed and focused it is, the better equipped you will be to do the delicate balancing act among budget, quality, administrative, and staffing concerns. Until you understand the dimensions of the problem, it is difficult to evaluate if the solution will work.

What different departments would potentially be involved in an improvement effort for timely delivery of food? As a manager you have to negotiate with other managers all the time. In this example, you might need to contact managers from Nutrition and Food Services or Pharmacy to develop an improved process for high-risk patients, and to put into place risk assessment policies, involving managers from Nursing Education and Internal Medicine, who would identify such patients.

The most successful improvement efforts involve a team approach, collaboration, and consensus building. Teams can cross departments or involve members of a single department. When struggling with prioritization issues, teams are most important so that expertise and objectivity are garnered from many sources. An additional advantage to teams is that when people become involved in a project, they feel more ownership of it and thus more commitment to its success.

Using a Prioritization Matrix

To wrestle in some coherent way with problems about prioritization, the NS-LIJHS Quality Management Department developed the prioritization matrix shown in Figure 3.2 specifically to help managers evaluate competing issues for performance improvement. The criteria are designed to assist managers in thinking through their priorities, reminding them to ask if the issue is a high-volume problem or one that regulatory agencies require be monitored. Does it conform to the stated mission and goals of the organization?

Potential areas for improvement are listed across the top of the matrix. Using a 0–5 scale to indicate minimum to maximum relevance, the team or the manager ranks each issue according to primary criteria. Is the issue related to high volume, one that affects a large number of people? Is the issue a high-risk process, one that poses safety threats to patients? Is the issue problem prone, so that without improvement, other problems will result? After evaluating each issue against the primary criteria, total the numbers. The maximum is 15

Selection Criteria		Issue								
		#1	#2	#3	#4	#5	#6	#7	#8	#9
Primary	1. High volume									
	2. High risk									
	3. Problem prone									
	Primary Total									
Secondary	4. Organizational priorities									
	5. Regulatory agencies									
	6. Benchmarking data									
	Secondary Total									
	Subtotal									
Tertiary	7. Patient and family needs and expectations									
	8. Risk management									
	9. Cost-effectiveness or resources required									
	Tertiary Total									
	Total									

Scale: 0= No Application   2= Weak Application   4= Strong Application
         1= Minimal Application   3= Moderate Application   5= Totally – Maximum Application

Figure 3.2.   Performance Improvement Prioritization Matrix.

and minimum is 0. If one problem is ranked higher than the others, it should be your top priority for spending time and resources to improve.

However, problems are often too complex to be neatly evaluated and categorized, and often you will not see an obvious, clear-cut problem that ranks much higher than others. In that case, continue the prioritization evaluation by adding the secondary criteria to the primary set. The secondary criteria involve the relevance of each issue to organizational priorities, the requirements of regulatory agencies, and the comparison of care via benchmarking data. Using the same scale, 0–5, each issue again gets a numerical value and these three are subtotaled and their total added to the primary total. Now the totals will range from 0 to 30. Those with the highest numbers should be targeted for performance improvement.

If no one problem is outstanding and further prioritization is required, you can use the tertiary criteria, consisting of evaluating the issues against patient and family needs and expectations, risk potential for legal action, and cost-effectiveness. What would be the cost impact of studying the issue, and can a case be made so that the administration will back the study and improvement implementation. Once the issues are quantified using tertiary criteria, the new subtotal should be added to the subtotal for primary and secondary criteria. The values will range from 0 to 45. The problems with the highest values should be studied. (If the numbers are still equal, reexamine the values placed on each item and recalculate them.)

Since you can't improve all processes simultaneously, making choices according to a matrix helps you define your priorities by quantifying one concern as more pressing than another. Quality management tools stress objectivity through deliberate, scientific, replicable, and communicable processes that can and should be used to underlie decision making.

The criteria established for our hospitals may not be relevant to you. If so, design your own set by developing criteria tailored to your particular concerns. Once you have useful criteria, rank order any problem or issue for its applicability to your selection criteria. Focus on the scope of care on which you have a direct impact. For an ED manager, for example, triage is crucial to ensure the appropriate flow of patients. On a neurological floor, discharge processes to another level of care for the postacute phase is important for LOS management. On a surgical unit, mobility and nutrition may affect patient recovery rates. In a psychiatric unit, the treatment plan and medication regimen may be most important in patient management.

To return to the ED example once again, your data might have identified several problems: patients were waiting a long time to be assessed and treated; many patients were leaving without being evaluated; patients who were released were returning within seventy-two hours; patients were leaving against medical advice; patients could not be moved to a floor because of delays in test results or lab reports; infection rates were rising. Which of these problems should an ED manager and staff address first? Using the matrix, your ED team would rank each identified issue for its relevance to the selection criteria, as shown in Figure 3.3.

You might rank excessive waiting time as a high-volume, high-risk, and problem-prone problem, and so enter 5 in the appropriate cells on the matrix, resulting in a total score of 15 out of 15. Fewer patients leave without being evaluated and therefore that problem is of moderate volume and gets a ranking of 3. But if a patient leaves the ER without being seen and is ill or in need of some kind of treatment or intervention, that circumstance could be a high-risk one, with a ranking of 4. Leaving without being evaluated could lead to other serious problems and so be considered problem prone, with a ranking of 3. The total of scores for this issue is 10.

You enter numbers in all the cells until one problem appears to have maximum relevance to most of the selection criteria. Figure 3.3 shows that—as often happens—there is no clear-cut conclusion regarding which problem to address after entering the rankings against the primary criteria. Both waiting time and laboratory turnaround have scores of 15, with infection rate close at 14. To make finer distinctions among the issues you are considering, move to the secondary criteria and enter numbers in the cells. Again the numbers are close, with no one problem particularly highlighted. Therefore, it is necessary to use the tertiary criteria. When the entire matrix has been completed, you see that laboratory turnaround time is most relevant to all the selection criteria. Your performance improvement efforts will then target making improvements in that process.

In addition to objectivity, another advantage to developing this kind of prioritization matrix is that it removes subjective value judgments. There is no right or wrong. You, as manager, and your team, rank each issue against predefined selection criteria. Priorities once

Emergency Department Selection Criteria		Waiting Time	Left Without Being Evaluated	Returns to ED Within 72 Hours	Left Against Medical Advice	Laboratory Turnaround	Increased Infection Rate
Primary	1. High volume	5	3	3	2	5	4
	2. High risk	5	4	3	4	5	5
	3. Problem prone	5	3	4	5	5	5
	Primary Total	15	10	10	11	15	14
Secondary	4. Organizational priorities	4	5	3	3	5	5
	5. Regulatory agencies	3	2	4	2	4	5
	6. Benchmarking data	4	4	4	4	4	2
	Secondary Total	11	11	11	9	13	12
	Subtotal	26	21	21	20	28	26
Tertiary	7. Patient and family needs and expectations	5	4	4	2	4	3
	8. Risk management	3	5	4	2	4	4
	9. Cost-effectiveness or resources required	3	1	3	2	5	3
	Tertiary Total	11	10	11	6	13	10
	Total	37	31	32	26	41	36

Scale: 0= No Application   2= Weak Application   4= Strong Application
         1= Minimal Application   3= Moderate Application   5= Totally – Maximum Application

Figure 3.3.   Performance Improvement Prioritization Matrix for Emergency Department.

established are not set in stone, however; they change with time and circumstance. Therefore, they must be reevaluated on an ongoing basis.

SUMMARY

Information based on quality data has the following characteristics:

- It is available from many sources.
- It promotes clearly defined goals.
- It reflects the expectations of the patients and the health care organization.
- It allows you to monitor care and target improvement efforts.
- It reveals compliance with regulations.
- It must be communicated to be useful.
- It should be related to outcomes and promote accountability.
- It can be useful in promoting change.
- It can be benchmarked against national standards to assess performance.
- It should be used to prioritize improvement efforts.

Things to Think About

- You are the manager of an ER and data reveal that an increasing number of patients are leaving without being evaluated, and that a high number of patients who are seen are returning within seventy-two hours.

  Keeping within your budget, you need to improve. How do you decide where to put your resources?

  Using the prioritization matrix, rank your quality concerns for your working environment.

CHAPTER FOUR

Managing Quality Data

W. Edwards Deming, a prominent quality theorist, is reported to have quipped: "In God we trust. Everyone else has to use data." The point here is that data are trustworthy, because they are objective. If you want to prove for yourself and your staff, or for your own manager, that the care you are delivering is good, what evidence would you rely on? Notions like *good care* and *quality* seem entirely subjective and based on individual judgment. What is good to you might not be good to someone else, or what is defined as quality care in one organization may not be so defined in another.

You could say, "Trust me, I'm doing a good job," or you could offer information, in the form of data, to objectively define an otherwise subjective concept. The best way to support your assertion that the care you deliver is quality care is to quantify your processes, services, and outcomes. With data, a manager can know if the staff is effective and efficient, and if patient outcomes meet expectations—of the manager, the patient, and the organization. Having data allows the manager to clearly communicate objective information about the delivery of care to other parts of the organization, or to administration.

Collecting quality data and analyzing that data for performance improvement is a complex process, one that frequently involves many steps and staff and requires time. In this section, we introduce some of the issues involved in gathering quality data and developing quality indicators for tracking performance. Some typical problems with the analysis and interpretation of indicators will be discussed as well.

GATHERING QUALITY DATA

The constant stream of information—about the daily activities on your unit, budgetary concerns, reports on employee turnover, sick leave, patient treatment plans, patient complaints, discussions of crises and crisis management, quality management reports on specific measures or processes, and reports from other services and divisions of the organization—that flows across your desk needs to be considered and interpreted to be of any use to you. If the information seems important to you and related to a process or service to which you give a high priority, you may want to drill down and investigate further. Therefore, when you have apparently relevant data, you start asking focused questions with the goal of gathering as much information as you can about a specific issue.

For example, you know that collecting data that tracks the movement of patients across the continuum of care and supports the coordination of services to promote an appropriate and timely discharge can lead to an appropriately short length of stay (LOS). If your LOS is high, it is your job to understand why and therefore you gather more data. Perhaps your inquiries reveal that most patients are discharged at around the same time, 11 A.M., and that leads to delays in cleaning some of the rooms and preparing the beds for new patients. You have identified a bottleneck resulting from a process—too many patients requiring simultaneous services—that influences the LOS.

Or imagine that you are a nurse manager and you hear about a patient on your unit who fell during the preceding shift. You recall several falls on the unit lately, but you don't really know how many times this has occurred or why or when because falls were not on your immediate radar screen. Perhaps you had a deadline to deliver a project and were busy with other concerns, or a different crisis required a great deal of attention. However, this new fall highlights the problem for you and you proceed to investigate.

Although investigation like this is necessary, it can result in other problems by disrupting the normal routine of work. However, if you anticipate disruption and plan how to deal with it, the consequences will be easier to manage. Also, the solution to the problem might result in new and costly services, with a correspondingly negative impact on your budget. You may need to provide one-to-one observation for a patient who is at risk of falling, for example, or redistribute the workload to allow for more intensive monitoring of one patient in a way that may lead to problems for other patients. As with any intricate and delicate construction, once you move one piece, the positions of others change, and unless you bolster the supports, the entire structure could weaken.

Regardless of the consequences, you realize that you need to analyze and improve the falls situation because falls are prioritized as a high-risk problem; they can result in fractures, surgery, or worse. Falls are also a patient safety concern, and since safety is a high priority for the organization, part of its stated mission, you prioritize the issue on your unit as high. Information about falls is available to you. You know the time, place, date, number, and reason for falls from the incident reports; you also are aware from the patient assessment and history and physical that certain patients are highly susceptible to falling. Falls have an impact on LOS, especially if they involve injuries that require tests and treatment. You learn that patients who fall, and their families, tend to complain about their care in a formal way, such as through satisfaction surveys or complaints to the organization, suggesting that better care would have prevented the fall from occurring. Patients and their families have instituted lawsuits as a result of falls.

With just a little thought, you realize that if you can understand the reasons for the falls on your unit and if you can implement some improvements that would decrease their incidence, you would be addressing the safety objectives of your organization, reducing the potential for malpractice claims against the hospital, increasing patient satisfaction, helping meet your budget goals, reducing LOS, and, most important, preserving patient safety—your primary charge as a manager. Therefore, you are determined to investigate and improve. In addition, you want to be able to assure your own manager or supervisor that you understand the problems in the delivery of care on your unit and that you can manage them.

Defining the Problem

To gather more specific information, you begin by asking your staff what they think might be the risk factors associated with patient falls on the unit. The wise manager knows that the frontline staff is a most valuable resource for data. If the answer is simple, say the floors are being washed frequently with something slippery at times when patients are apt to walk on them, and the situation can be rectified with a phone call to Housekeeping, great. The problem is easily solved.

Generally, however, problems are not so quickly resolved, and you will require further investigation. If your staff cannot pinpoint a solution, your next step is to form a multidisciplinary team to try to brainstorm what could be the reasons behind the falls. Remember, as a manager you don't have to have all the answers, but you do have to ask the right questions of the right people.

To arrive at some understanding of how extensive the problem is, you may want to count falls over a given period. Once you have that data, you will need to evaluate if the number suggests that falls are a very serious problem on your unit or not. How will you determine this? As manager, you want to be able to compare the care you deliver with the care delivered on other units. Is your unit particularly subject to falls? If there is a difference between your unit and a comparable one in relation to the number of falls that occur, what could be the reason?

It may also be important to identify when the falls occur, throughout the day or only in the middle of the night shift, and to identify if patients who fall have any characteristic in common. Is the age of the patient relevant or is a particular diagnosis associated with falls? Or a medication? Under what circumstances did each fall occur? Was there a lack of response to the call-bell when the patient needed to go to the bathroom?

The more you ask, the more you know. You realize that you need additional information to answer these and other questions and to pursue some of these lines of inquiry. Use data sources that are readily available to you: daily census reports, information about staffing ratios, nursing and physician notes regarding patient condition, end-of-shift reports, and so on. As a manager, you have access to a great deal of information, including the patients' medical records.

The medical record can be a gold mine of information about the services rendered to patients—and their effectiveness. It will also describe the tests and medications each patient received as well as outcome and discharge disposition. Medical record information is also used to gather aggregated data about hospital performance. The medical record, as the source of payment for the hospital, needs to be as complete as possible. Coders read through the medical record to construct a bill based on the information therein.

In addition, many other sources of information are available to you. You can easily find data regarding nursing staff numbers and patient-staff ratios. The Quality Management Department may collect data about the number of falls throughout the hospital that you can use to compare the incidence on your unit with others. Risk Management may have data available about any malpractice claims that have been filed as a result of falls. Nursing may have data about any injuries that have occurred. There may be external databases that you can tap as well.

All this information might help you better understand the situation and evaluate how critical your problem is. When you start collecting information in a focused way, with a question to answer (why are patients falling?) or an assumption to test (older patients fall at night), you are involved in gathering quality data.

The primary reason you ask questions and gather quality data is to evaluate if any corrective action should be taken to rectify a situation, and what that improvement should be. If your inquiry determines that the patients who fell were sedated, perhaps the prescribing physician and Pharmacy staff need to be part of an improvement process. If patients fell and injured themselves during shift changes, then you might have to assess the modes of communication and procedures for coverage during this vulnerable time. You can't determine if improvement is necessary until you know the causes, dimensions, and scope of the problem. In other words, you can't manage until you measure. The analysis should lead to the development of a fall-prevention program, and measurements should be developed to assess the effectiveness of the improvement.

Information is key to performance improvement, so you need to collect data specifically tailored to what you want to improve. If you don't focus your data collection efforts, you may end up with a great deal of general information that sheds only shadows on your issue, rather than light. For example, is every fall of interest to you, or only those falls that result in injury to the patient? Do you want to concentrate on any special time period, such as falls that occur during the night shift, and collect data only on that? Perhaps you want to focus your improvement efforts on a specific group of patients, such as those who have diabetes. Or you may want some combination, and target your data collection to patients with diabetes who fall during the night shift and whose falls result in injury. In other words, before you start collecting information, determine the general or specific dimensions of the issue you are investigating.

Determining the Scope of the Problem

After carefully defining the problem you want to address in terms that incorporate an implicit assumption or an idea that you want to test, you can take a count of the number of patients who meet the specific criteria you have developed. However, a simple count or raw number, although interesting, may not be informative enough for you to decide if improvements are necessary. Say you learn that over the course of a week (or a month) ten of your patients have fallen, how would you interpret this piece of information? Is that a reasonable number to expect to fall, a situation that, although unfortunate, you could tolerate as normal in the delivery of care, or would that number be an indication of a very serious problem?

To decide if this number is acceptable, you may want to compare the number of patients who fall to the total number of patients on your unit. If you have ten patients who have fallen in a week, and your unit has only ten patients on it, that's an indication of a bigger problem than if you have ten patients who fall over the course of a month out of a hundred patients. Therefore you want to know not only how many patients fall but how many fall compared to the number of patients you have who might have fallen, or who had the opportunity to fall, and over what time period.

To better understand the scope of your problem, then, you want to know what percentage of your patients have fallen during a specified time period, which will reveal more about the process of care than a simple raw count. A percentage is a fraction; therefore calculating a percentage allows you to capture information both about the incidence (how many) of falls in the numerator, compared to the number of your patients who might have fallen, that is, who had the opportunity to fall, in the denominator. If you have ten falls per thousand patients (1 percent), over the course of six months, perhaps you would determine that your improvement efforts should be focused elsewhere. But if you discover that every week your unit has ten falls per fifty patients, or 20 percent, you know you have a far more serious problem to address.

You need both a sense of the dimensions of the problem, that is, data that reveal how many incidents were related to how many possibilities, and also a time frame to delimit that data, to help you measure, or *quantify*, some aspect of the care you are delivering.

Defining Numerators and Denominators

Using percentages or rates to assess and monitor care forces you to carefully define what you are investigating. For example, if you decide to examine only those falls that resulted in hip fractures in diabetic patients over seventy years old, that population would define your numerator. Or if you are interested in determining the effects of medication on falls, you might collect data on the number of falls that occurred to all patients on sedatives (or any other medication); then that number would be your numerator. Defining the numerator results from asking a specific question, such as how many patients fell while taking sedatives, or from making an educated assumption, such as that diabetes and age influence falls in elderly patients.

Once you determine what you want to study and know the characteristics of your numerator, you need to carefully define the population from which you want to collect that information. The way we think of developing such measures is that the numerator consists of the number of events—falls or whatever is being studied—that occur, and the denominator consists of all the opportunities where that event could have occurred. If you are investigating falls that result in hip fractures in the elderly, your denominator might be the number of patients on your unit who are over seventy years of age. If you are trying to determine if medication (sedatives) has an impact on falls, your denominator would be the total number of patients on sedative medication (see Figure 4.1).

The Role of Indicators

When you define, collect, and examine quantifiable information with a purpose in mind—for example, to understand the number and type of falls on your unit—you are involved in establishing quality indicators.

Indicators *indicate*. A meat thermometer indicates the temperature of the meat, a ringing telephone indicates that a call is coming in, and the rising or falling stock market index indicates the vagaries of the

$$Rate = \frac{Numerator}{Denominator} \times 100$$

$$Quality\ indicator = \frac{Events}{Opportunities}$$

$$\begin{array}{l} Rate\ of\ hip\ fractures \\ from\ falls\ of\ patients \\ more\ than\ 70\ years\ old \end{array} = \frac{Number\ of\ hip\ fractures\ from\ falls}{Number\ of\ patients\ over\ age\ 70} \times 100$$

$$\begin{array}{l} Rate\ of\ sedated \\ patients\ who\ fell \end{array} = \frac{Number\ of\ patients\ on\ sedatives\ who\ fell}{Number\ of\ patients\ sedated} \times 100$$

Figure 4.1.   Defining Indicators.

economy and the monetary value of your stock. Indicators all around you signal information about your environment. Quality indicators indicate whether or not the quality of care being delivered is good, excellent, or poor.

A manager who attempts to manage without benefit of quality indicators is a manager working without the essential tools of the trade. Even if the information revealed is problematic or unpleasant, you need it. Unless you monitor care via indicators, you are hiding your head in the sand. You won't be informed if clinical or financial issues need attention if you are to meet your own expectations or those of the leadership of the organization. You may not be aware of the educational needs of your staff. Your patients may be vulnerable to adverse events or incidents. Indicators serve as an early warning system for problems.

ANALYZING DATA FOR PERFORMANCE IMPROVEMENT

If you examine a quality indicator such as the rate of falls at one point of time, you have a single data element. But one data element offers insufficient information on which to base any conclusions about the care processes. Even if you think your rate of falls (or whatever you are examining) is high, with only one data element, you don't know if that number represents a fluke and is a single occurrence or if it reveals a pattern or trend that bears watching and correcting. You need to track an indicator over time, usually three months—a quarter of a year—to determine if you have a trend.

Establishing Databases

By collecting and tracking quality indicators over time, you are establishing a database for that indicator. With a database, you can quantify the experience of care and make intelligent decisions about performance improvements. If, then, you determine to implement any changes, such as a fall-prevention program or a one-to-one observation policy, continuing to track the indicator on the database will reveal whether or not your changes have been effective and have made an impact on the process of care. Certain indicators, such as falls, should be monitored on an ongoing basis, given today's patient population. As the percentage of patients who are elderly and enter the hospital with multiple health problems increases, the risk for falls increases as well.

The database should be used to monitor progress, illustrating where you are, compared to others, regarding a specific indicator, and where you want to be. National standards and benchmarks are available in the clinical literature, and you can establish thresholds to define excellent care. If your data show that you have not reached the acceptable threshold for a period of time, you may want to introduce improvements or evaluate the interventions introduced to reduce the rate of falls.

Quality indicators are sometimes calculated as an index rather than a rate or percentage. An index is simply a fraction, with the same defined numerator and denominator as the corresponding rate, only multiplied by a thousand rather than a hundred. The reason you collect data and develop databases is to evaluate performance and target improvement efforts. Using an index rather than a rate may be appropriate when you are measuring a phenomenon with very few occurrences (for example, patient suicide). If you have very few incidents, it is difficult to determine if you have a problem. An index helps you normalize chance occurrences when the numbers are small.

Figure 4.2 charts the falls index of seven units within a hospital over a one-year period, illustrating the variation in the number of falls. Each unit's index can be compared to the system benchmark of 2.5. The database indicates that your unit, G, has the highest incidence of falls in the hospital. Therefore you target falls for an improvement effort.

Once you have defined your quality indicator—and perhaps established a database to track that indicator over time—you require still more information before you can determine what kind of improvement needs to be implemented. Since your database reveals that the falls rate

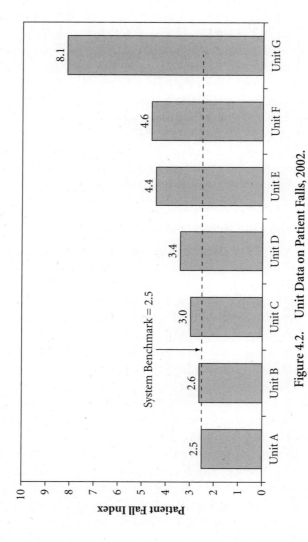

Figure 4.2. Unit Data on Patient Falls, 2002.

on your unit is unacceptably high, much higher than comparable units at your institution, you want to know what factors are contributing to this situation. In other words, you need to further analyze your data.

It may be useful to know the demographic variables of your patients, including such factors as diagnosis, age, sex, date of the fall, time of day when the fall occurred (that is, what shift), whether or not an injury occurred and if so, the nature of the injury, or if the patient was in restraints. Information about these variables may help you analyze the factors that contribute to the outcome of falls, that is, you might see a relationship, or a *correlation*, between falls and one of these variables. Each of these factors can be measured and then they can be displayed together as shown in Table 4.1. The resulting table of measures may suggest relationships among the variables for further investigation. Information may also indicate which other departments or services should be involved in the improvement effort.

Exploring Relationships

Your goal is to understand the situation and the processes involved with the large number of falls on your unit. Table 4.1 charts demographic and clinical information regarding twelve patients who fell during a single month. Look for commonalities. Present the data to your staff during your supervisory meetings. Such an exchange will promote ideas about the relationship among indicators.

Table 4.1 reveals no obvious relationship between falls and any particular diagnosis, nor age (although the range is more elderly than otherwise), nor sex. However, more falls occurred at night than at any other time, and more occurred in the bathroom than anywhere else. The falls resulted in injuries to all but one patient.

You might assume that the use of restraints would eliminate falls, and indeed the reason patients were restrained might be that they had been assessed at being at risk for falls. But the data indicate that this is not the case; in fact, those patients who were on restraints had more severe injuries than those patients who were not restrained. Your database might lead you to investigate the relationship between falls and restraint usage.

As you make improvements, you should be able to monitor their effectiveness through these interrelated indicators. For example, you might be able to look for any indication that the rate of falls decreases when the night shift has an educational program regarding falls, or

Patient	Diagnosis	Age	M/F	Date of Fall	Shift*	Location	Nature of Injury	Restraint Yes	Restraint No	LOS
1	Diebetes Mellitus	76	F	5/01	D	Bathroom	Bruised Arm		X	5.0
2	Heart Failure ·	81	F	5/03	E	Bathroom	None		X	5.9
3	Myocardial Infarction	63	M	5/03	N	Hallway	Bruised Leg		X	4.3
4	Community Acquired Pneumonia	83	F	5/04	N	Next to Bed	Broken Hip	X		15
5	Diabetes Mellitus	72	M	5/10	N	Bathroom	Head Stitches		X	8.5
6	Hip Fracture	77	M	5/10	E	Room	Subdural Hematoma		X	7.1
7	Gastro-Intestinal Bleed	63	M	5/15	D	Bathroom	Stitches—Arm		X	5.5
8	Lung Cancer	65	M	5/18	D	Room	Broken Hip	X		8.5
9	Hysterectomy	62	F	5/21	E	Next to Bed	Broken Arm	X		4.3
10	Prostate Cancer	69	M	5/22	E	Hallway	Bruised Leg		X	6.6
11	Leukemia	79	F	5/25	N	Bathroom	Stitches—Arm/Leg		X	18
12	Psychosis	79	M	5/30	N	Bathroom	Subdural Hematoma		X	15

Table 4.1. Patient Fall Data, Unit G: May 2003.

*Key: Shift D = day; E = evening; N = night.

restraints are eliminated in favor of increased monitoring. You may want to train staff to do more frequent rounds on patients on medication that increases disorientation and that might also increase their urgency for using the bathroom. Staffing effectiveness is about more than simple numbers and ratios; staff has to be used appropriately to address patient needs.

You should be wary of making hasty conclusions, especially if you don't spread the net widely enough and include multiple indicators. You don't want to suggest correlations and relationships without data as support. Regulatory agencies are now asking about staffing ratios and the composition of the staff whenever an incident occurs. They recommend that hospitals and health care organizations correlate human resource indicators such as staffing ratios with quality indicators such as falls. A common suggestion that makes a kind of intuitive sense is that patient falls are related to the number of nurses and other health care staff available for bedside care on the unit, if deployed appropriately.

When the NS-LIJHS tracked staffing ratios with the rate of falls, at first glance there seemed to be no correlation between them. Our conclusion was that a single indicator (that is, staffing) was insufficient to explain so complex a phenomenon as falls. For example, case mix index—that is, the degree of illness associated with specific diagnoses—in combination with staffing ratios, may be more informative about patients at risk for falls. Keep peeling the layers until the explanation for the fall makes clinical and administrative sense.

Interpreting Indicator Data

Some indicators, like the rate of falls, may be established because you have collected information about a problem on your unit, but not all indicators are developed on a unit or service level. You might be asked to collect information and monitor processes because regulatory agencies dictate that you report information about them (for example, reporting sentinel events such as providing care to the wrong patient). Or the leadership of your hospital may determine that certain indicators should be analyzed because it will help the organization evaluate resource allocations such as utilization of specialty beds.

Some indicators should be measured in real time, that is, *concurrently,* when the patient is in the hospital and during follow-up care after discharge. Infection rates should be monitored concurrently to alert you to any adverse outcome such as a surgical wound infection.

Other indicators can be examined *retrospectively*, that is, by looking backward; for example, readmission rates can be derived from an examination of medical records. It is important that you understand how to measure the quality indicators reported or required throughout the organization.

Whether concurrently or retrospectively analyzed, the value of data is in the interpretation. If the readmission rate is high, or increasing, you have the opportunity to implement different improvements and then monitor whether or not the efforts have made an impact. For example, you could attempt to make changes in the discharge process and see if the data reflect any change in readmission rates, or you could investigate if something in the medical or nursing management of the patient should be changed, implement improvements, and then track the indicator to evaluate effectiveness. You might want to examine patient and family information about posthospital care to assess how that influences readmissions. The point is that you want to use your data for performance improvement.

Another traditional quality indicator concerns skin integrity. Skin ulcers or pressure injuries, also called *decubiti* (and once upon a time "bed sores"), are thought to reflect the quality of bedside nursing care because with proper care, these injuries can be minimized or eliminated. Nurse managers collect these data to monitor the delivery of nursing care, as does Quality Management staff. Since skin ulcers can result from prolonged exposure to the bed surface, nurses are expected to rotate bedridden patients frequently and massage the skin to avoid this problem. If skin ulcers appear, the nurse can order specialty beds and special ointments.

Skin damage is not difficult to monitor and recognize, and it is incontestably an indicator of care, having an obvious impact on patient wellbeing. Health care organizations that don't address this issue are marked as problem organizations by the CMS because skin ulcers are perceived as conditions that can and should be eliminated. If decubiti are not caught and treated early, complications—as extreme as gangrene—can be quite serious; therefore daily nursing care and vigilance are crucial.

Tracking the rate of decubiti requires that the nurse count the number of patients who develop skin ulcers in the hospital and report those data to their manager for collection. If the unit manager or a member of the Quality Management staff who monitors the rates of skin ulcers, notices that the incidence is increasing or decreasing, the unit manager can ask why, and implement appropriate interventions or establish standards for best practices. Remember, the primary purpose of measuring a clinical phenomenon is to change behavior and to increase safety for patients by introducing improved processes in the delivery of care.

Accountability

But nothing is simple in health care. Typically, nursing staff report data on skin ulcers or pressure injuries to unit managers who in turn report the data to the assistant director of Nursing. In the NS-LIJHS, unit managers report information to the Quality Management Department, which is responsible for aggregating the data for the hospital and system. Quality Management calculates trends in the data over time for different units and departments and reports the information back through the quality staff to the managers and to the nurses on the unit. It can't be stressed enough that information has to be communicated to be useful. Collecting, and even analyzing, is not enough.

Several years ago, while compiling and monitoring the data on pressure injuries, the system Quality Management staff realized that there had been a steady rise in both the incidence and the severity of decubiti across the entire continuum of care, from the medical units through nursing homes to home care. This is a high-risk, high-volume problem, affecting 9 percent of all hospitalized patients and 23 percent of long-term care residents, according to a report by the Agency for Health Care Policy and Research, with estimated costs for treatment nationwide well in excess of $3.5 billion annually. The health system ranked this problem as a high priority for developing process improvements.

Policies and processes to deal with skin ulcers had been developed and approved years before. Cute gimmicks including paper clocks had been introduced into several ICUs to remind the nurses to turn their patients every ten minutes. However, these clocks were found to be dusty and yellow from lack of use. Defining the correct process, and even having reminders in place to reinforce it, does not ensure that the correct process will be followed. We found that even with detailed policies, care was being delivered idiosyncratically depending on the training and experience of the nurse and not on any objective basis.

If a patient develops a skin ulcer, it is easy to cast blame on the unit nurses. However, nursing managers, who are responsible for nursing education and orientation, are also culpable; if a good assessment process is in place, those patients who are at greater risk for developing skin ulcers can be carefully monitored. Disciplines other than nursing have to be involved in skin care as well. Nutritional assessment is important because skin integrity can be influenced by diet. Physical Therapy also should be part of the care process, as the condition is exacerbated by lying in bed and not moving. Skin damage can develop if a patient undergoes lengthy surgery; therefore Surgery, Recovery Room, and Critical Care unit personnel need to know about skin care issues. Pain management has to be incorporated into the patient care plan because skin ulcers are frequently painful and require medication. Therefore pain management staff and the Pharmacy should be part of the skin care team since decubiti may require special medications and ointments. Specialty beds need to be ordered through the Purchasing and Materials departments, so they have a stake in skin care also. Because the elderly are particularly vulnerable to skin ulcers, a geriatrician might be part of the multidisciplinary team formed to develop processes to care for the patient with decubiti. Diabetes also makes patients more susceptible to skin irritations, and so Internal Medicine staff may be involved.

Convinced that skin care is not a simple nursing issue? One of the reasons quality indicators like the rate of skin ulcers are useful to different managers is that almost any department can be among those implicated in the process of care as well as patient outcomes. This multidisciplinary involvement is one of the reasons that Quality Management Departments generally report quality indicators throughout the hospital or even the system. The complexity of modern health care services is so interdependent that it is a rare process that can be considered in isolation.

Defining the Concept Under Investigation

If you, as a manager of any of the involved departments, receive data alerting you to a rise in skin ulcers on your unit, how would you interpret that information or understand what the information means? Before you can begin to answer that question, you need to know the definition of a "skin ulcer." Even if a concept or condition seems obvious, definitions can vary widely. Does the term refer to skin redness (how red?) or a deep lesion in the skin (how deep?), or to something or everything in between? Who determines the meaning?

Clear definitions are crucial or there will be no way to ascertain if everyone who is supplying the data is reporting on the same phenomenon the same way. Before reliable data can be collected and analyzed, then, a standardized definition needs to be established and then communicated throughout the hospital or system. The person or group responsible for the definition needs to be identified, and the organization needs some sort of rationale or basis for the derived definition. You might not imagine that an indicator like falls or pressure injures could be defined in various ways, but multiple definitions are always possible. Without an explicit definition that is communicated throughout the system or organization, people can end up with the medical equivalent of comparing apples and oranges because the indicator just specifies "fruit that is round" instead of what is really of interest.

When the NS-LIJHS Quality Management Department determined to standardize the definition of a pressure injury so that uniform measurements could be collected and monitored for all units throughout the continuum of care, the first step was for the staff to research the relevant clinical literature from medical and nursing journals and communicate with experts in the field regarding issues of definition and indicator development. Using research and clinical expertise can help to validate the definition, which is especially important when competing definitions might be chosen.

Skin condition can be extremely subjective and not at all easy to quantify, unlike body temperature, which can be quantified, as can a rise in blood pressure, sugar levels, and so on. But if a patient has some redness and tenderness, how does a nurse quantify "some"? The Quality Management group determined that we needed to reduce subjectivity as much as possible and find a reliable and objective scale for clarity because the more objective a definition we could develop, the less risk of variation in the reporting of this indicator we would face. Also, with an objective definition, uniformity and standardization of reports are much more likely.

Research revealed that such an objective assessment tool for predicting pressure sore risks, accepted within the health care community to assess skin integrity, could be adopted for our use across the system. Using this scale would enable caretakers from various units and services to define and monitor quality statistically rather than impressionistically. But again, it is important to remember that simply determining the best process does not ensure its implementation. An educational program, including teleconferences and in-service training on the use of this tool, was necessary before the nurses became comfortable and familiar with it. Since the scale would be used by different raters at different times to guide clinical decisions, everything possible was done to ensure uniformity of use. In time, we were able to feel secure that the data collected were reliable, uniform, and meaningful.

If you want to manage well, you need to measure well. The value of standardizing definitions for measurements cannot be overstressed—without uniform, clearly defined measures, it is impossible to collect reliable data, and without good data, it is difficult to make reasonable decisions about performance improvement, staffing needs, physical and financial resources, and so on. Even a phenomenon as seemingly straightforward as falls requires careful and thoughtful definition.

For example, does a fall occur whenever a patient stumbles, or does the patient have to end up on the floor? Does a patient fall if a caregiver is assisting with a move into a chair or onto a bed or is a fall something that happens when a patient is alone or unattended? How is the level of medication implicated in a fall, that is, if a patient is unstable because of medication and collapses on the floor, should that be defined as a fall? Should patients on certain medications require restraints so that they don't fall? What, then, is the relationship among restraint use (another quality indicator), sedation, and falls? Many indicators have similar issues regarding definition. It is not that one definition is superior to all others, only that agreement itself is essential; everyone involved has to use the same definition for the data collection to be reliable and complete. That's the only way you can be sure that you are measuring exactly what you want to measure for improvement.

However, even when you carefully define your indicator, other issues with data collection still need to be addressed, especially in defining exactly what should be reported or included in the measurement. For example, if a patient has more than one pressure injury, should that be counted as one or more? If a person has two pressure injuries and one is improving and the other is not, which severity should be reported? If the patient arrived on the unit with a skin ulcer that perhaps occurred on another unit, should that be counted on your unit or the other? Careful definition of the indictor clarifies the numerator. One knows to count, for example, only one pressure injury per patient, even if there are multiple sores.

Determining the appropriate denominator is also problematic and (like everything else) requires thoughtful definition. We said that the denominator of a quality indicator should be calculated as the opportunity for a certain event to have occurred. Say that it has been established that the numerator for reporting rates of skin ulcers should be the number of patients who have one or more pressure injuries.

(Notice that we are counting patients rather than injuries. If we wanted to count injuries, the definition would be different, and refer to the number of injuries, regardless of whether or not they were on the same patient.)

What would be the most appropriate denominator, giving us the most information about the process of care? Perhaps a reasonable denominator for decubiti should be the number of patient days (opportunities for the patient to acquire a pressure ulcer), which can be tracked from the hospital database. If patient days are used, what period of time should be delimited?

Count all the patients on the unit who developed pressure injuries during one month, and make that number a factor of the number of patients who could have received pressure injuries, that is, the number of patients who were on the unit during that month. What about transfers? Some patients who present at the beginning of the month will move off the unit to another floor before the end; should they be counted? Or think about opportunities for falls. Should falls be counted over the number of patient days, or the number of patient beds on the unit, or over some time period? Measurements require a great deal of thought and planning.

Another traditional quality indicator is return to the ED within seventy-two hours. If patients are returning so quickly, it may be because their care wasn't adequate the first time around. ED managers, hospital administration, nurses, and Resident Education and Quality Management staff, among others, find this indicator of quality care informative. One can count the number of people who return to the ED, but what should be the denominator? Should the denominator be calculated as the number of admissions to the ED within a specified time period, or rather should it be discharges during that time period, say a month? If you think about it, you realize that a patient cannot return to the ED unless already discharged. Only then would the patient have an opportunity to return. But what about the patients who are discharged within seventy-two hours of the last day of the month? They wouldn't be counted because they would return at the beginning of the next month.

You see how challenging definitions and calculations can be. You must always take into account your objective in determining what you want to study. If you want to show that the rate of patient falls is low, you may use patient days. If you want to show that the problem is big and needs improving, you choose the number of patients who fell.

Many care providers are reluctant to involve themselves with measurement. Measurements require time and attention. Because measurements reveal the successes or failures in a process of care, the effort leads to accountability. Problems are identified—whereas without measurements they may be ignored. We have found that developing carefully defined indicators is worth all the trouble because measurements are key to improvement; problems don't disappear by themselves but through being addressed by means of a deliberate methodology.

Making Improvements

A quality indicator, tracked and trended over time and communicated appropriately, is worth a thousand words. That is to say, an indicator, if carefully defined and reliably collected and reported, reveals facts about care that are very hard to refute. Good data can promote improved clinical practice and influence and even change cultural values.

For example, a patient's LOS can be tracked for clinical appropriateness, as determined by national databases. If the LOS is longer than the national standard, whether due to complications, inefficiency, or inadequate care, the cost to the institution may increase, using money that might be spent elsewhere more productively. Doing a good job is cost-efficient. Having appropriate resources to devote to care improves quality. Quality and cost are interdependent in health care.

Imagine a situation where the data at your institution (or your service) indicate that the LOS is higher than the national average (data are available for comparison). Administration wants to reduce it since a high LOS indicates inefficient services and overuse of resources. Physicians are reluctant to participate in any LOS reduction effort, saying that their patients are sicker than the national average and therefore their LOS is perfectly appropriate. But LOS data can be broken down into smaller and smaller data elements, from the hospital, to the service, to the unit, to the specific physician.

If one doctor or unit has a higher LOS than others with a similar patient population, it is possible to tease out the variables that explain the extra time. Comparative data can be used as most compelling evidence. If the physicians see data showing that patients with the same diagnosis as theirs and with the same comorbidities have a shorter LOS everyplace else, they might be willing to agree to make changes in their practice.

Improvement efforts are best spurred by data. For example, when the administration noticed that a unit at one of the system hospitals had an LOS almost double what was predicted (by the CMS) as typical for that patient population, Quality Management staff collaborated with the professional staff on the unit to analyze the process of care. Until the LOS data pointed a finger at the efficiency of the unit, staff had been unaware of any problems. After a detailed investigation of the medical records of the patients on the unit and an analysis of how patients were moved through the delivery of care process from admission to discharge, the investigators realized that the unit had an unrecognized bottleneck regarding assessment and documentation for physical therapy (PT).

That bottleneck was having a major impact on increased LOS. Patients who had physical therapy appropriately triggered by the nursing assessment had an LOS of 4 days, while patients who did not have PT appropriately triggered by the assessment had an LOS of 13.5 days. By sharing the results of their investigation and analysis, quality management and the staff on the unit devised new procedures to improve the triggering of PT with great success. In this example, LOS data were used to great advantage, resulting in changes that improved care for the patients, who had a shorter hospital stay, as well as an increased revenue for the institution because resource utilization was improved and unnecessary expenses were reduced. Data helped change behavior.

SUMMARY

Objectifying care through quality indicators has the following features:

- It promotes standardization and uniformity of care.
- It enables care to be quantified and communicated.
- It defines problems for performance improvement efforts.
- It is the result of a team effort and multiple departments.
- It requires carefully defined measures (numerator and denominator).
- It involves defining the scope of the problem within a time frame.
- It can be tracked and trended over time.
- It can be displayed on a database.

- It enables comparisons.
- It reflects the effects of improvements and changed behaviors.
- It can be concurrently or retrospectively examined.
- It enhances interpretation and analysis.
- It increases accountability of the caregiver.
- It improves clinical practice.
- It provides the organization with information crucial to resource allocation.

Things to Think About

- You are a unit manager and it comes to your attention that a number of your patients have fallen, with serious consequences.

  What questions do you ask?

  What information do you collect?

  How?

- You are a Food Service manager or an Infection Control supervisor, or are in charge of the environment.

  What quality indicators would you develop to track the value of your service?

  What would be the numerators and the denominators?

- For your own service,

  Define your own opportunity.

  Define the event.

  Develop your own quality indicators.

CHAPTER FIVE

Using Quality Tools and Statistical Methods for Data Analysis

—∿∿—

O nce you gather relevant data, you need to analyze it to make informed and intelligent decisions about your services and about performance improvements. Through the analysis of data, you can determine whether or not you are meeting your objectives, and if you are not, your data may indicate which processes should be further examined. Although most health care organizations have financial analysts and Information Technology departments geared toward measurement and quality coordinators who collect, manage, and analyze data, the ability to interpret data independently offers great advantages to any manager or supervisor.

If you can assess processes quickly and effectively, you are less dependent on the time constraints and work requirements of others. Statistical tools, which many managers may not be familiar with and may even be wary of, are so useful for understanding and organizing information (data) that we want to introduce some of the basics in this chapter. These tools, combined with quality management methods, provide managers with the means to address and communicate about problems and outcomes, to manage crises, and to standardize care through reducing unwanted variation.

UNDERSTANDING THE PROBLEM

To return to the example of falls, say the patients on your unit have congestive heart failure (CHF) and are generally over seventy years old. Information reported to you reveals that the number of falls on your unit is higher than in the rest of the hospital, and you propose to investigate why this situation should exist. You collect information about the problem and devote time in your weekly staff meetings to developing ideas about solutions. To form a study and improvement team, you identify the stakeholders. In addition to the floor nurse, you bring in Housekeeping (floors), Materials (call-bells), Risk Management (injuries), Pharmacy, and a geriatrician.

You ask all these specialists to offer data from their fields of expertise that might shed light on the problem of falls. Housekeeping staff can collect data regarding time of cleaning, their cleaning responsibilities, and any safety precautions they take during cleaning. Materials Management gathers data on equipment that could be potential obstacles for patients navigating around the room and hallways. Since patient satisfaction surveys describe poor response to call-bells, Nursing can collect data regarding response time, time of day, reason for call, and so on. Pharmacy has data on medications that can lead to confusion and disorientation. Risk Management has data on patient injuries that result from falls. The geriatrician can examine the different data sets with patient falls to explore any correlations. The group meets over time, as long as necessary, to investigate the processes involved and to recommend improvements.

Cause and Effect

Every patient fall is an event and can be analyzed for cause. It may be useful to carefully examine a single instance of a problem, here a specific patient fall, to locate weaknesses in the delivery of care. If weaknesses are identified in one case, you can assume that they would be implicated in other cases, and that the process should be improved.

A cause-and-effect diagram (sometimes called a fishbone diagram or an Ishikawa diagram, named after its inventor, Kaoru Ishikawa) is a useful tool to illustrate the various factors that have an impact on a particular outcome, in this case, a patient fall. A fishbone analysis can help the team identify the root causes of a problem, especially a complex problem. The assumption underlying such an analysis is that many factors contribute to an outcome, some more salient than others, and that these factors can be organized into distinct categories. Once you have detailed the possible causes of the poor outcome, you want to cluster the causes into categories that define the large "bones" of the diagram.

Figure 5.1 shows a cause-and-effect analysis of a patient fall. The major categories that contributed to this adverse outcome involved characteristics of the patient, issues in the environment, hospital policies, particulars of the equipment, and the personnel involved in caring for the patient. Another situation may have alternate categories. This patient's diagnosis, CHF, required a diuretic for medication; a diuretic increases urinary output and so may contribute to a greater urgency for toileting. Greater urgency for toileting may make the patient try to get out of bed without assistance. In addition, this patient had a history of falling and an unsteady gait. All these factors should have alerted the staff to this patient's risk of falling.

The environment also contributed to the fall. It was cluttered and poorly lit; the call-bell was out of reach and the floors may have been slippery. Under the heading of policies, the performance improvement investigative team determined that assessment was poor and thus implicated in the outcome, and that although a fall-prevention program had been instituted, not all personnel had been adequately trained. The equipment available to the patient was also deemed to be a factor, especially inappropriate footwear and a faulty bed alarm. The health care staff involved in the patient's care also contributed to the negative result, not only the nurse and physician, who were responsible for educating the patient about the environment and assessing the patient's condition for risk of falling, but also the aides who responded (or not) to the call-bells, the physical therapists who helped provide the patient and family with information and techniques regarding mobility, and even the patient's family, who might have left the environment in a way that put the patient at risk, for example, not returning the side rails to the upright position.

Some of the identified factors can be manipulated and improved, others cannot. Obviously, nothing can be done about the patient's age, medical condition, or history, other than take note that they may be contributing factors. However, you can manage and improve other aspects in the care process, such as the poor lighting and the lack of proper assessment, or the disabled bed alarms and the inadequate access to the call-bell. Improvements may involve repairing equipment,

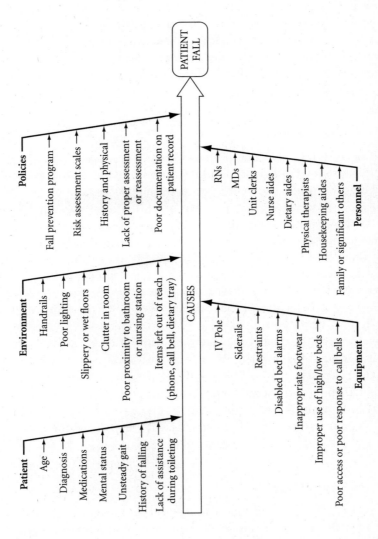

Figure 5.1. Cause-and-Effect Diagram: Patient Fall Analysis.

identifying who is accountable for ongoing monitoring and maintenance, or educating staff for improving assessments. Until you have analyzed the problem and organized the causes intelligently, you don't know what improvements are necessary.

Locating weaknesses in the delivery of care leads to targeted improvement efforts. We have found that using data to relate process to outcome can resolve or minimize problems over time. For example, increasing staffing does not necessarily reduce the incidence of falls. However, educating staff about patient safety and a fall-prevention program may do so.

Flow Chart

Another tool that has value in describing a process is a flow chart, which diagrams the sequence and decision points in a process. This tool helps to outline the major points in the process and can reveal bottlenecks, redundancies, and ineffective or inefficient elements. You start the flow from the beginning (top) and detail every step of the process until the end. Figure 5.2 is an example of a flow chart for determining how a hospital should report an adverse event.

The first consideration is to establish if the event caused harm to the patient. If yes, then a multidisciplinary team is convened to review the case and to determine if the standard of care was met. If no harm occurred to the patient, then the event is tracked over time and reported through the quality management committee structure so that staff is alerted to the problem. If the standard of care was found to be met, then the issue travels through the structure. However, if it was not met, then reports should be made to the appropriate agencies. The report is communicated to the hospital quality committee and the medical boards. Once the event is analyzed, the result of the investigation is reported back to the hospital medical boards.

Run Chart

A run chart is a line graph that can be used to understand trends or patterns over time. If, for example, you wanted to track Emergency Department (ED) visits during a month, a run chart might show you the peaks and valleys of the number of people who require care, and during which time periods. Figure 5.3 illustrates the number of ED visits that occurred during a one-month period. The horizontal or X-

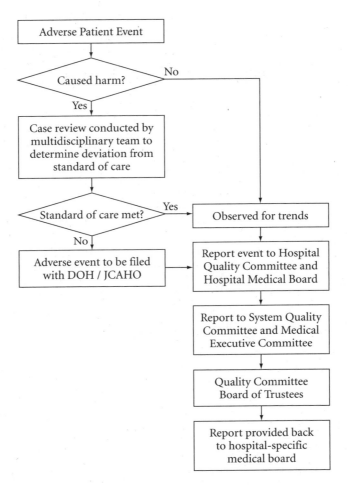

Figure 5.2.   Flow Chart: Reporting Adverse Events.

axis is labeled with the day of the week, and the vertical or Y-axis records the number of visits to the ED.

Looking at this graph, it becomes immediately apparent that ED visits rise on weekends, Saturdays and Sundays, for each of the four weeks charted. This easily gathered piece of information may well have important consequences for the manager responsible for staffing on weekends, or for Radiology and other services that may be under-staffed on weekends. Gathering objective data bolsters your case if you are requesting resources or revising existing policy.

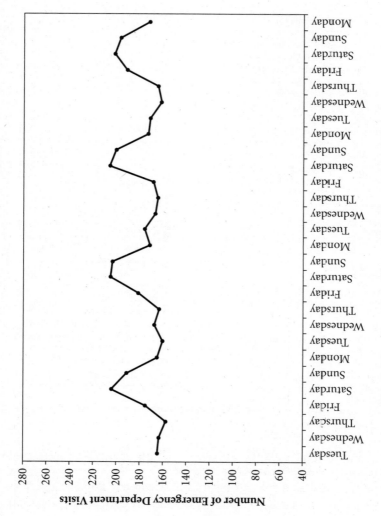

Figure 5.3.   Run Chart: Emergency Department Visits.

DESCRIBING INFORMATION

Once you have collected data about your service or process, you want a way to describe it so that you can understand and communicate a sense of what your findings illustrate. Data can be quantitative, that is, numerical. Weight, cholesterol, and sugar levels are examples of quantitative information. Not every kind of data is numerical, however; some, such as patient satisfaction or quality of life, is categorical (related to categories). Regardless of the type of data you are analyzing, a first step in describing your data might be identifying the average of your distribution—the value that best represents the entire set of data.

Knowing the average is useful because it gives you a value that best represents an entire group of data elements. An average reflects information about what is typical about your data; think of it as a kind of quick summary.

There are three basic ways to characterize a distribution, depending on the information you are looking for: the mean, the median, and the mode. Each measure contributes a specialized piece of information about your data.

Mean

The *mean* identifies the typical value in a range of values. It is calculated by adding all the values in a group and then dividing the resulting sum by the number of values in the group. For example, when school students try to anticipate the grade they will receive in a class, they add up all their test grades in the relevant time period and then divide that score by the number of tests they took. Or, to say it another way, you take the sum (the Greek letter sigma, written as Σ, is used to mean summation) of the values you are interested in and divide that number by the number of values (n) in the group. Sometimes the mean is symbolized by M.

Say you had five tests in a course and received grades of 95, 90, 90, 85, and 45. (Well, you had a bad day!) Your mean score (M) is 95 + 90 + 90 + 85 + 45. The sum Σ of those scores is 405, which you divide by 5 (the n) to give you a result of 81, a B–. You know that the grade of 45 is pulling down your average (mean) score. If you never took that test and you only had the other four grades, your mean score would be much higher, 90 (95 + 90 + 90 + 85 = 360; 360 / 4 = 90), an A–.

The score of 45 is distorting—referred to as *skewing*—the data set. The mean is sensitive to extremes or *outliers* in the data (like that 45).

Or say that you are collecting information about the blood sugar levels of one of your patients. Over the course of a week, your patient's morning glucose test results are very variable—120, 112, 90, 145, 132, 101, 161—and you want to know the mean for the week because the patient is supposed to increase medication if the average for the week is more than 120. By calculating the mean, you find the week's average reading is 123; therefore you know to institute the appropriate treatment.

Median

When you want to know what is typical about your data, and not have the result skewed by the outliers, you can calculate your average another way, by identifying the *median*—the midpoint in your data set. The midpoint means that 50 percent of your data points lie on one side of that value and 50 percent on the other side. Thus, the median is not affected by the extremes or outliers that skew the mean.

For example, for many managers, the LOS of their patient population is important information. But LOS data are easily skewed. Patients admitted to rehabilitation tend to have a high LOS and so skew the data in one direction; patients who stay only twenty-four hours skew it in the other. To understand how to reduce LOS, you need to analyze what is normal, and that means knowing what is most prevalent in your population. You want information about those values that cluster around the median, rather than any extremes.

To calculate the midpoint, organize your data so that the numbers fall into a sequence—low to high or high to low—and then simply count up or down to see what is in the middle. If you had eleven patients on your unit and you wanted to calculate the median LOS, and their LOS was 6, 3, 7, 16, 2, 4, 3, 6, 8, 1, and 19 days respectively, you would order the numbers from low to high—1, 2, 3, 3, 4, 6, 6, 7, 8, 16, 19—and find the midpoint in the series. In this data set, the median is 6 because five values are lower than 6 and five are higher. If you have an even number of data points, find the two in the middle and calculate the mean of those two numbers to get the median.

You can see that calculating the median involves a different process from calculating the mean. And, in many cases, these different processes yield different numbers. Think about blood sugar readings. If another of your patients has blood sugar readings that are 120, 116, 132, 117, 103, 112, and 190, the mean (or average) would be127, but the median 117. You wouldn't want to start medication for high sugar (over 120) without more information. In this case, the median is a more representative average than the mean because it accounts for the skewing effect of the extreme data point of 190.

Mode

Sometimes it is informative to know the value that occurs most frequently in a set of data. That is the *mode,* which is useful especially in describing a high-volume population. The mode differs from the mean and the median because, unlike the mean and median, the mode can represent data that are categorical rather than quantitative. For example, to find the most frequently occurring condition in your patient population you would want to use the mode. If twenty patients on your unit have pneumonia, ten patients have CHF, and forty patients have diabetes, the modal condition would be diabetes, because that is the most frequent condition. The number forty is not the mode, it's just how often the modal condition occurs in that group. If every value has the same number (ten pneumonia, ten CHF, ten diabetes), then there is no mode. If the two greatest values occur the identical number of times (ten pneumonia, twenty CHF, twenty diabetes), the distribution is said to be *bimodal,* or if more than two, it is called *multimodal.*

The measure of central tendency you choose to calculate depends on your goal—what you want to describe. The mean is what most people think of by *average,* but you are better off to use the median when extreme data points skew the data and make the mean misleading. Use the mode when you are interested in qualitative or categorical data such as disease process, eye color, or sex rather than the numerical values for those categories.

UNDERSTANDING VARIABILITY IN DATA

In addition to the commonalities and general tendencies of your data, it may also be informative to understand something about its variability—how different the data points are from each other (remember that test score of 45). For example, the set of scores 7, 6, 3, 3,

1 shows some variability. Another set of data, 3, 4, 4, 5, 4, has the same mean (that is, 4) but less variability. The set 4, 4, 4, 4, 4 has no variability at all, although it has the same mean as the others. Therefore, knowing the mean alone may not be descriptive enough of the extent or range of your data.

Range

If you want to know the *range* of your data, which means how widely spread the data points are from each other, subtract the lowest number from the highest. The result is the range. If during the month of September the temperature varied from 50 degrees to 80 degrees, the range of temperature variation would be 30 degrees (80 − 50 = 30). In the example of blood sugar noted in the discussion of the median, the range would be 74 (190 − 116 = 74), which reveals a wide dispersion.

Standard Deviation

The range gives you some sense of the big picture, but it is very general. Often you might like a little more information regarding the range, a kind of fine-tuning that would tell you how far away from the mean, on average, a set of data points is. You can calculate this by calculating the *standard deviation* (SD). That's what SD is, the average distance from the mean. The larger the SD, the farther the average data point is from the mean. The formula illustrated in Figure 5.4 may look very complex, but it's simple enough when you take it apart (and calculators and computer programs do most of the work for you). Understanding the formula, even in theory, is not a bad idea, since people in health care services tend to talk about standard deviation.

The formula instructs you to do a series of operations in a specific order. Since what you are examining is the variation from the mean, you first calculate the mean. Then subtract the mean from each individual score (X − X-bar). Then square that result (to get rid of negative numbers). Add together (sum) all the squared deviations from the mean and divide by one less than the total number of data points ($n - 1$). Take the square root of that number (since you squared the sum of the scores you have to now unsquare them, or take the square root). The result is the SD. Computers and calculators make finding the SD quite manageable.

$$S = \sqrt{\frac{\Sigma \ (X-\overline{X})^2}{n-1}}$$

Where: S is the standard deviation

Σ (sigma) tells you to find the sum of what follows the symbol

X represents each data point

$\overline{X}$ (called X-bar) is the mean of the data set

n is the number of data points being analyzed

Figure 5.4. Standard Deviation Formula.

If the SD is 2.5, it means that the data points are, on average, 2.5 units of the variable being studied away from the mean; if the SD is .4, then the data points average only .4 units away from the mean and the data are much more uniform. The greater the SD, the greater the difference among the values, and this gives you information about the variation in your data.

You will be able to determine if the data are normal in terms of a particular characteristic. For example, if you have wide variation of LOS from the mean, that is, a large SD, it might indicate that your patient stay is very long or very short (distance from the mean in either direction) and needs to be studied in comparison to the average population. Using this tool, a manager can look beyond a single instance of a problem and assess patterns and trends.

Bell Curve

When you plot data variability on a graph, the resulting line tells you a great deal about the data. If there is no particular lopsidedness in the data, it will look like the *bell curve* illustrated in Figure 5.5.

A bell curve, or *normal distribution*, is perfectly symmetrical—high in the middle and trailing off evenly to both sides. Many phenomena are normally distributed: blood sugar levels, body temperatures, height of the population. Extremes are rare (which is why they are called extreme) and fall at the ends of either side of the bell curve. The middle of the curve, where most of the results are, represents the average (the mean, median, and mode). Interestingly, almost all normal distributions fall

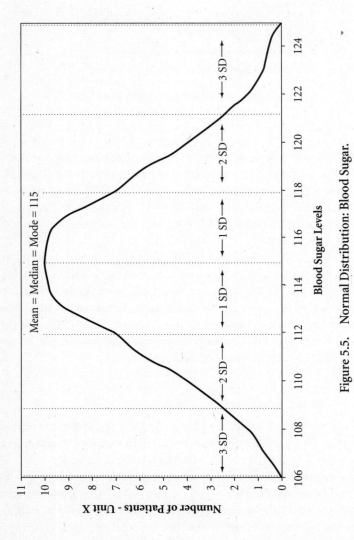

Figure 5.5.   Normal Distribution: Blood Sugar.

into the value of plus or minus 3 SDs from the mean. Therefore, if you know the mean, and the SD, you can compute 3 SDs in each direction from the mean on a graph. Normal data will fall within this range.

Bell curves are useful to graphically represent large sets of data. If you observe ten patients with pneumonia in an effort to determine when medication is—normally—switched from intravenous (IV) to oral (PO), you might not be successful because that small a group could easily have too much individual variation. But if you examine the experience of a hundred or a thousand or ten thousand patients, the norm would be more reliably identifiable. The larger the data set, the more reliable the average and the more normal the distribution. Generally, in a normal distribution, 1 SD from the mean includes 34 percent of the values. That means 68 percent of all values fall between −1 and +1 SD around the mean.

USING DATA TO IMPROVE CARE

Describing your data by identifying the average and the range and variability of the data points is a good place to start. But because you will want to use the data to interpret the processes involved in your delivery of care and improve performance if necessary, you might want to use your data to ask—and answer—theoretical or research questions based on the objective facts revealed by the data.

Hypotheses and Variables

Research begins with a *hypothesis,* which is a theoretical explanation or assumption that may account for a set of facts and that requires further testing to prove if it is accurate. Generally, the goal of the hypothesis is to investigate the relationship between certain characteristics, events, or factors and to assess the impact, if any, they have on each other.

Any characteristic, event, factor, attribute, quantity, or phenomenon that can have different values is called a *variable.* Often you may be interested in determining how one variable can predict or influence another. For example, you hypothesize that the greater the number of falls on your unit, the longer the LOS on your unit will be. The underlying assumption of this hypothesis is that patient falls prolong LOS. You hope to investigate the relationship between these two variables, falls and LOS. In this case, you want to explore the possibility that falls (the independent or predictor variable) contribute to LOS (the dependent variable).

Null Hypotheses

The starting point of your research is to posit the *null hypothesis,* which serves as a standard against which you can measure your results. You assume that no relationship exists among the variables you are investigating. Formally, the null hypothesis might be: there is no relationship between patient falls and LOS. That's your starting point—zero connection. Until you have proof, that is, objective evidence of a relationship or correlation between these variables, you assume that any relationship that you might see is due simply to chance.

Research Hypotheses

To test the relationship, you develop a research hypothesis that posits a relationship between the variables. Such a statement might be very general, stating something as simple as "patient falls are related to LOS." Or it can be highly specific, something along the lines of "if patients fall and sustain serious injury, they will require services that will prolong LOS."

Your research hypothesis is based on what you are interested in, and your experience; it is an educated guess, which is not the same as an idea taken from thin air. That is, it would be possible but not particularly useful to say that people who eat pizza twice a week in their twenties will develop diabetes when they are eighty, if they have not ice-skated every Thursday. If, astonishingly, your data indicated some such relationship, you would be hard-pressed to explain it. A more educated hypothesis, based on experience, would be to say that people who eat carbohydrates at every meal might require more insulin than those who eat primarily protein.

Sampling

Once you develop your hypothesis and define your research question, you need to formulate a method to test it. Testing your hypothesis can present logistical problems. Time and money are usually limited, so collecting data on every single instance of the phenomenon you are investigating can be unrealistic, not to mention overwhelming.

Although it might be ideal to monitor the dietary issues of every one of your patients, it may not be feasible. What can you do? The way researchers resolve this issue is to collect data on a sample, a portion or subset of the population or of the occurrences in question and then make inferences from the results. If you take a sample from the population you wish to study and carefully formulate a hypothesis and test it on that sample, you should be able to generalize the results to the entire population.

For example, some businesses gather information about the television-watching practices of the general population. How do they know which shows are most popular? They can't require every person watching TV to report what they are watching all the time, or monitor the viewing habits of the entire country, so they choose a representative sample, a small number of people they think have characteristics similar to the larger population (economic background, ethnicity, age, gender) and track the TV shows those people watch. From the results, they generalize to (make inferences about) the total population.

You want your research sample to closely resemble the population you are studying. If your interest is male patients over sixty-five with hip fractures, you collect data on a sample of that highly specific group. But you might want to investigate how everyone or anyone might respond and not limit your inquiry to any group; to do this, you choose a sample population at random (unsurprisingly called taking a "random sample"), such as the third name on every tenth page of the phone book or every tenth chart on your unit over the past thirty days.

INTERPRETING RESULTS

How do you test your hypothesis? You formulate your question and define your sample population. Then you collect data over an appropriate time period—at least three months. In our experience, less than three months of data collection is insufficient to reveal a meaningful trend.

Significance

Once you collect your data and discover a relationship among variables, you need to evaluate the quality of the relationship. You might have heard the term "statistically significant" used about data. The expression means that the variables you are connecting to one another are indeed meaningfully related and the patterns you see are not simply the result of chance. Researchers measure the significance level of what they are testing (again, you can use computer software that calculates this easily) and report something as having, for example, a $p < .05$. That means that there is a one in twenty or 5 percent ($.05 = 5$ percent) chance that the relationship between the variables you are testing is merely the result of chance.

Here's an example from the ICUs. Some units have full-time intensivists and some don't. You want to explore whether or not there is a relationship between the presence of a full-time intensivist and the rate of "self-extubations," or patients who remove their own ventilator tubes rather than have the tube removed by a care provider. The null hypothesis states that there is no relationship, that the rate of self-extubations in units with and without intensivists is identical. The research hypothesis posits that patients in units with an intensivist have a lower rate of self-extubations than those patients in units that have no intensivist. You identify your sample population, in this instance patients from units with and without intensivists, and collect data over time about the self-extubation rate (after carefully defining the numerator and denominator). If indeed you find a difference between these two populations, how can you determine whether or not the result is due to what you think it is? That is, is the presence of the intensivist what makes the difference, rather than another characteristic such as the amount of sunlight on the unit or the quality of the nursing care?

The level of significance provides information about how likely it is that you have made an error, the wrong assumption. Generally good research results tolerate a .05 error rate, or a 5 percent chance of having made a spurious or erroneous connection.

Interpreting Meaning

However, if your data show a statistically significant result, that doesn't mean that the results are meaningful to you, only that they are not the result of chance. Many other variables about the issue, that is, the context, need to be taken into account before changes should be instituted. For example, how expensive is it to have an intensivist and what other services might be affected? Can an educated nurse or a respiratory therapist fulfill the same role, perhaps less expensively? As a manager, you need to use your data intelligently, as a springboard to understand the issues you wrestle with every day: services and re-sources. In today's economic climate, especially, decisions cannot be made without good data. Lack of data can lead to inappropriate investments, or the over- or underuse of important interventions.

Displaying Data

Sitting alone with your data will not improve the delivery of care in any way. To be useful, data must be displayed and communicated. You may well be familiar with several visual representations of data: charts, tables, pie charts, bar graphs, line graphs, and so on. Using these visualizations for data reports is effective in allowing people to quickly assess what is going on. The ideal choice depends on the type of information or data you have and the purpose of the analysis or communication in progress.

LINE GRAPH. A simple line graph can be used to reflect trends. For example, a manager who was concerned with the number of patient falls on her unit collected data for a year and summarized the data using a line graph. Figure 5.6 tracks the number of patient falls on the Y-axis over time, which is represented monthly on the X-axis. The graph revealed a sharp increase in the number of patient falls during the month of June. Although the data showed this increase and alerted the manager to a potential problem, it did not supply any explanatory information.

TABLES. The manager who was worried about falls on her unit had the good sense to track demographic information about her patients as well as the raw data on how many fell in each month. She collected monthly information about patient age, LOS, number of falls, and so on, and posted it to a spreadsheet, which is a sort of table. (See Table 5.1.)

A table (or a spreadsheet, which can be computer-generated) gathers a great deal of information in one place and is most useful for comparing data of different types. It allows you to present and analyze multiple factors simultaneously. The additional information revealed by Table 5.1 provided an explanation of the data presented in the line graph because it showed that in June the average age of the patients jumped from the early and mid-seventies to almost ninety. With this added information, she determined to investigate the relationship between increased age and falls. Often, having access to different

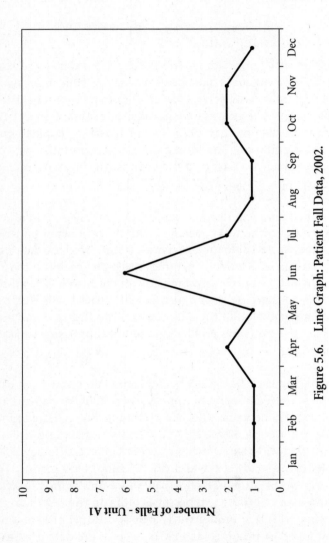

Figure 5.6.   Line Graph: Patient Fall Data, 2002.

Month	Age	LOS	Number of Falls
January	70.38	3.05	1
February	74.10	3.71	1
March	73.32	3.85	1
April	71.13	4.20	2
May	76.10	3.90	1
June	89.99	4.99	6
July	75.59	4.10	2
August	70.35	3.87	1
September	72.23	3.20	1
October	74.39	4.23	2
November	71.10	4.12	2
December	70.80	3.99	1

Table 5.1.   Table or Spreadsheet: Patient Fall Data, 2002.

kinds of data in different formats suggests areas for investigation that you would miss if you relied solely on a single display.

BAR GRAPHS. When the data are discontinuous, that is, consist of distinct or different categories, then a bar graph, column graph, or histogram may be the most effective display. Figure 5.7 is a bar graph displaying the LOS for patients with different types of insurance.

The X-axis identifies the insurance carriers, and the Y-axis identifies the frequency or numerical value of the average LOS. The data summarized in this figure show that Medicare patients have a higher average LOS (eight days) than that of patients who have either HMOs or private pay-for-service insurance.

PIE CHARTS. A pie chart can illustrate how various factors fit into a larger picture. Figure 5.8 shows the disposition of all the patients of one hospital.

At a glance you can see that the majority of patients (79 percent) who leave the hospital go to home or self-care. This visual information allows the unit managers and also the hospital administration, social workers, and discharge planners to better prepare for discharging patients.

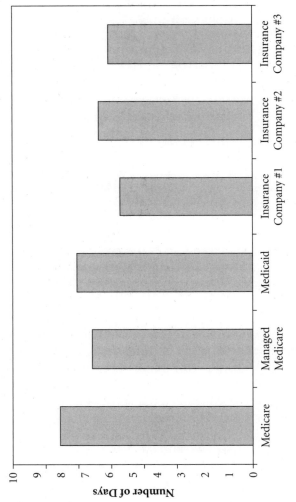

Figure 5.7.   Bar Graph: Hospital Length of Stay by Insurer, 2002.

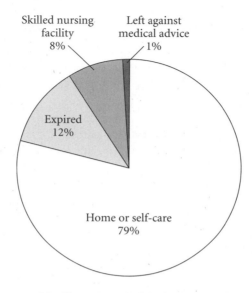

Figure 5.8.   Pie Chart: Hospital Patient Disposition, 2002.

MONITORING PROCESSES

Data analysis must be an ongoing process because you want to be sure that the care you are delivering remains at a consistently high level. How do you know that some process is consistently stable and working well?

For example, consider postoperative wound infections. One of the reasons you collect data on this is to ensure that the infection rate stays relatively stable and very low, not one month a rate of 2 percent and another 5 percent. If your rates remain within certain expected parameters, between 1 percent and 2 percent a month, you can assume that nothing special or peculiar has influenced the process. It is under control.

But what if one month you have 7 percent rate of patients with wound infections, and the next month 6 percent and the third month 10 percent? At that point, you might want to investigate what is responsible for these seemingly erratic numbers. The health care industry has been accused of underreporting poor quality care, and low rates of infection tend to be a result of underreporting rather than improved quality. Therefore, it is important when you see a disparity in data to find out if the reporting system has changed, or if there has been an educational effort to encourage increased reports of problems and errors.

Control Chart

A useful quality tool that is designed to monitor the stability of processes is the control chart. A control chart is similar to a run chart (the chart that tracks a process), but a control chart contains upper and lower limits on either side of the process average to warn you if the process you are monitoring is out of control, or not stable. The chart will reflect this by showing data points that cross the boundary (upper or lower) limits. One aberrant data point might be a result of chance or of some unusual occurrence, but if you see three or more data points that cross the boundary, it is usually a good idea to investigate the cause of the variation. In other words, a control chart helps you quantify variation, distinguishing between normal and abnormal levels.

How do you distinguish normal from abnormal variation? The first step is to record data over several months and determine the mean average for the process you are analyzing. Every process includes some normal variation, and therefore it is important to know what is normal before you start analyzing what is not normal, or is a problem. As an alternative, if you feel that waiting to collect data over months would endanger your patients or otherwise be problematic, you can do a *retrospective analysis,* using data from preceding months or years, and derive the mean average from what has happened in the past.

Remember that normal variation is usually distributed in the shape of a bell curve, and that almost all data points fall within three standard deviations (3 SDs) from the mean. If you turn the bell curve on its side, you can establish the upper and lower control limits of 3 SDs from the mean. However, health care institutions generally want more consistent processes than the typical bell curve allows. They compute upper and lower control limits as only 1 SD from the mean, as shown in Figure 5.9, because the less variation from average, the tighter the process.

To develop a control chart, collect data over time. Experts suggest at least fifteen data points are necessary for the control chart to be meaningful. Calculate the mean and the SD. Figure 5.9 shows the number of postoperative wound infections over the course of fifteen months, with a mean average of 3.13. You can set the upper and lower control limits more or less broadly, depending upon how much variation in the process you can tolerate.

Once you determine your upper and lower limits, you carefully track any data point that lies beyond those limits. If you begin to see

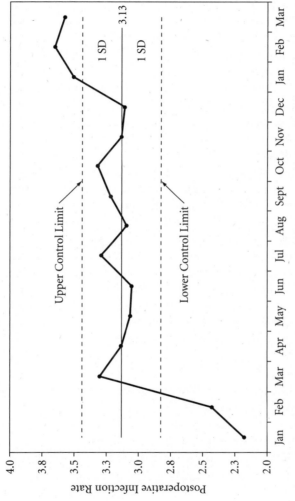

Figure 5.9. Control Chart: Postoperative Wound Infection Rate, January 2002–March 2003.

that your process is out of control, usually by recording three or more spikes in either direction beyond the limits, you need to investigate why. That's when you collect your team for a focused review, and if appropriate, begin a PDCA cycle.

You can be flexible about establishing upper and lower control limits, and you can use information other than standard deviation to set the limits. For example, say that the LOS on your unit is high, as much as fifteen days. In other similar units, the LOS for a comparable patient population is only seven days. This information is available in the administrative databases that your Information Services Department can provide. You can use a control chart to watch the data associated with LOS, establishing nine days as the upper limit, and seven days as the mean, and perhaps four as the lower limit. It may be that the national benchmark for your situation is lower still, three days, but you have a long way to go. A more reasonable goal may be to lower your LOS not to seven immediately, but to eight, then down by fractional days. You can keep tightening the control limits around the established mean until your goal is reached.

While collecting the data (remember that you need to watch a process for at least three months) you do your analysis. How is your unit different from the others in terms of patient mix, availability of physical therapy for ambulation, nutrition for special diets, and so on? If there is no difference in the age, sex, ethnicity, or comorbid conditions in your patient population, why is there a discrepancy in their LOS? In the caregivers? In some process? Using the PDCA you can begin to make improvement interventions based on the information you have accumulated and use the control charts to monitor your improvements.

Performance improvement strategies are not only used for problem resolution. You can take a process that is running adequately and try to improve it. A good manager does that: asks constantly if there is room for improvement. And there always is. By asking the right questions of the right people (staff, focus groups, experts) you will be able to use information to evaluate and improve the care you deliver.

SUMMARY

Managers can use these tools and methods to understand, communicate, and display information about problems and outcomes:

- A cause and effect analysis categorizes various factors that have an impact on an outcome.
- A flow chart diagrams sequences and decision points in a process.
- A run chart displays trends over time.
- The mean average identifies the value typical of a data set, but is affected by extremes in the data, whereas a median average is not.
- The mode differs from the mean and median average because it can represent typical categorical values.
- Determining general tendencies of data, with the range and the standard deviation, is useful in understanding variability.
- A bell curve illustrates normal distribution of data.
- Data can be used as a basis for research.
- The null hypothesis posits no correlation between variables, whereas a research hypothesis posits a relationship.
- Research can be conducted on a sample or a subset of the population under study.
- Statistical significance calculates the degree to which correlations are the result of chance.
- Data can be displayed in tables, charts, or graphs, depending on what information is to be communicated visually.
- A control chart is used to monitor a process to see if it is in control and to focus attention on any aberrations that require further investigation.

Things to Think About

- Patient satisfaction survey data regarding your service vary greatly for the different areas addressed in the survey: perception of nursing care, staff attitude, food quality, team communication, noise level, room condition, and education about the disease process. What tools would you use to interpret the data?
- How would you display the results of the data analysis to your manager?
- How would you display the results of the data analysis to your staff?

CHAPTER SIX

Translating Information into Action

Information is knowledge, and knowledge is crucial to effective management. Without knowledge, decisions are based on flimsy supports, whereas good decisions, grounded in data, result in improved care—which is what you want. Data can provide an early warning system, alerting you to problems or disruptions in the delivery of quality care. Without such an alarm, your service remains vulnerable to crises and your patients are at risk. With data, you have the underpinnings of measurements that help you evaluate your performance on a continual basis. This ongoing monitoring of your service keeps you apprised of how well your unit is performing. You certainly don't want to be in a position where anyone—your manager, or someone in Administration or Quality Management—informs you that your service or unit is performing poorly, that you are managing badly, and that your patients have complained.

Good managers are not caught by surprise. They are the first to know, fully conversant with the problem and right on top of it. You should be the one to notify your manager, or whoever is most appropriate, that your data analysis has revealed an issue regarding the care you are managing, and that, having investigated the dynamics of the problem, you have the outline of an improvement initiative. Good data, good decisions, good care.

Any improvement initiative has to take into account the interdependence of services and disciplines so critical to the delivery of seamless quality health care. Therefore, managers have to understand more than the issues related to their own service; they also have to appreciate the impact of their services on other parts of the organization. The interrelationship implies that any change that is instituted to improve performance on one unit will have an impact on many other services as well. One of the advantages of quality management methodology is to encourage a unified and integrated approach to care throughout an entire organization.

PLANNING FOR IMPROVEMENT

The quality management methodology for performance improvement is deliberate and careful. As we have repeatedly stressed, it never makes sense to rush in and start reacting to situations without having a carefully thought-out plan of action. If you simply respond to problems as they occur, you won't be able to address their underlying causes or take steps to prevent similar problems in the future. Imagine the work involved, for example, in analyzing every individual fall as it occurs, filling out the incident report, trying to educate your staff to avoid a similar event, assuring Risk Management that you have safety procedures in place, and explaining to the patient's family what happened and why. Performance improvement always involves change, and change involves planning—deliberate, careful, data-driven planning.

Identifying Problems

Potential problems surface when the data you are using to monitor and evaluate the processes of care alert you to them. For example, in an organization committed to a short length of stay, if data show that your LOS is increasing, it may be a sign of a problem. Patient complaints about your service could also identify a problem, especially if three months' data reveal a sharp increase in complaints over preceding months. Cues come from all over the health system regarding how you are managing care. If, for example, you manage a radiology unit and data reveal that turnover time is so long that physicians can't proceed with care, then improvement is necessary. Or bed turnover data might reveal that your unit is taking a much longer time than similar ones to admit new patients. Any issue related to patient flow through your unit might also indicate a problem—admission, treatment, medication—that requires investigation and improvement.

But improving care is not limited to problem solving. Improvement is always possible—and desirable. If you manage to get your LOS down from seven days to six days, that is an improvement. If you further reduce your LOS to five days, you would be improving resource consumption still further. Or if you implement a new program and your data reveal you have 85 percent compliance, you can work toward 95 percent or even 100 percent.

As you think about initiating improvements, list the factors in the delivery of care that you believe are the most essential to a successfully managed unit. Ask yourself what the overall purpose of your department is, and how that purpose interacts with the services delivered in the rest of the hospital. For example, if one of your primary purposes is to ensure patient safety on your unit, then you plan to provide patients with an environment that is clean and in compliance with infection control protocols. Information about cleanliness is available from other disciplines. You might request input from the Infectious Disease Department about appropriate procedures, as well as from the nurses on the unit who will be responsible for monitoring conditions to see that those procedures are being followed appropriately.

To get a sense of the impact of cleanliness on health, you might ask the safety officer or the Risk Management Department about accidents or claims against the hospital that were initiated because of something in the patient's environment related to the condition of the patient's room. Housekeeping might offer you insight into what factors are involved in keeping the rooms clean. With this information in hand, you can develop a database of relevant indicators such as the rate of infection or compliance with sterilization procedures, and over time this will help you quantify the care you deliver. If data reveal any disruptions in the process, you know what to investigate.

Proactive Improvement

Data collection and improvement efforts should be proactive as well as reactive. Obviously, when you discover a problem or a poor outcome, you have to take steps to deal with it and improve processes so that the problem is reduced or eliminated entirely. Even without a problem, however, if you identify an aspect of care that you would like to see improved, you can and should implement change and monitor the improvements. A third route to improvement is to identify potential problems and work to correct them before they reach the patient.

How can you identify a problem before it ever occurs? One way to do this is to collect data on *near misses*—occasions where something almost went badly wrong, as when two airplanes inadvertently come within a few feet of each another. A near miss is an accident waiting to happen; next time the conditions arise, whatever prevented the harm might not intervene. Your staff will have some idea about the risk points involved in the delivery of whatever service they render. Without thinking, when members of a health care team recognize a potential danger to a patient, they take steps to minimize the risk. Nurses who catch themselves about to administer the wrong medication (or the wrong dosage) to a patient (or the wrong patient) will stop and automatically correct the problem. Transport team members who realize that the name on the transport order does not match the name of the patient in the bed will stop and make further inquiries. If a diabetic patient is served a tray full of inappropriate food, full of sweets, and someone, either the patient or a family member, realizes it, the tray is taken away and Nutrition is informed. In other words, potential errors are corrected frequently and so instinctively that they may not even be recognized as danger signals.

However, bringing these near misses to consciousness through collecting data about them is a tremendously useful way to identify areas of care that should be assessed. Near-miss data reports make staff highly aware of the risks in their environment and processes. The difficulty is in acquiring the data. On a busy unit or service, when the workload is heavy, stopping to fill out a form about an accident that could have happened if it wasn't averted may seem unproductive, a waste of precious time. Part of the manager's job is to convince the staff of the importance of bringing this information to light, with the very real possibility that a tragedy could be averted.

Imagine that an inexperienced nurse is about to hang an IV with a medication that needs to be diluted, assuming that the Pharmacy would have taken care of anything required before delivering it to the floor. A second nurse happens to glance over and realizes that the incorrect, and perhaps lethal, dose is about to be administered to a patient. The second nurse of course stops the process, and the first nurse gratefully corrects the error. Both nurses continue their work without reporting this near miss.

The next day another new nurse makes the same mistake, administers a drug without diluting it, but this time no one stops the error from occurring. The patient has an adverse reaction, perhaps even dies. This devastating occurrence could have been prevented if the staff had been alerted to the potential for danger. If a mistake can happen once, it can happen again. By reporting near misses, staff increase patient safety and help avoid errors. When people understand the value of recording near-miss data, they are willing to take the time.

However, it is not solely time constraints that prevent the reporting of near-miss errors in most organizations. There is the more subtle problem of culture, where health care workers are reluctant to admit that they may have endangered a patient, been incompetent, or simply done something stupid. Peer pressure to be perfect is powerful, and people are often ashamed to admit to mistakes. Therefore, it is up to the manager to create an environment where staff is not embarrassed to admit potential errors, but on the contrary realize that the well-being of the patient is at stake if they do not.

Changing the habits of a lifetime is an enormous challenge. At our system, we have instituted educational sessions about the value of near-miss reporting and developed anonymous forms so that no individual name is attached to an error report. In one institution, rewards are given to the unit that reports the highest number of near misses because leadership recognizes that reporting potential problems is the most effective way to keep serious events from occurring. Near-miss reports are circulated through the quality structure so that every unit is able to learn about potential hazards wherever they appear. In a patient-centered environment, near-miss data help identify opportunities for improvement.

THE PDCA CYCLE FOR PERFORMANCE IMPROVEMENT

Once a problem has been defined and you have determined that a process should be improved, how do you go about fixing it? The methodology that we have found most productive for monitoring and improving performance is the Plan-Do-Check-Act (PDCA) cycle. The cycle is continuous, repeating itself again and again, with no beginning or end, and plenty of overlap among the stages (see Figure 6.1).

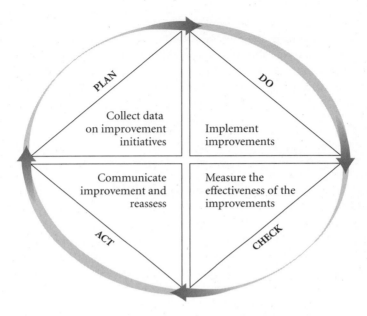

Figure 6.1. Performance Improvement Methodology.

The PDCA process involves planning for change or improvement constantly, and prioritizing and reprioritizing your improvement efforts based on carefully defined measurements and whether or not the problem involves high-risk, high-volume, or problem-prone processes, and if it dovetails with the goals of the organization (P). Improvements are implemented (D) while collecting data about the problem or process under investigation, and checked through ongoing data analysis (C) to evaluate whether or not the change has had the desired effect. Then the improvement is implemented, refined, or rejected, and if successful, communicated and introduced throughout the organization (A).

This methodology is so productive because it relies on basic common sense to understand a process that affects outcomes, uses data as the basis for increasing knowledge and developing process improvements, evaluates the improvement over time, and standardizes the improved processes for a high level of quality.

Because improvements most often include learning new habits of behavior, the PDCA cycle enforces and reinforces deliberate learning and strategic change. Imagine what is involved in learning to play chess, or change a tire, or program a VCR. First the learner has to have the desire to acquire the new information or skill, then fundamentals about the process have to be discovered. The new skill has to be practiced, with the expectation that mistakes will happen, but that one can learn from mistakes as well as from successes. Increased knowledge, real improvement, and changed processes require a great deal of time and patience. There is simply no quick fix.

Take Time

Yet time is such a valuable commodity for health care workers that a manager may feel pressured to hurry up and change. In the long run, however, the time spent in carefully developing good processes is far less than the time required for reacting to individual problems, each of which, until resolved, can derail or disrupt the delivery of services to patients. Integrating the PDCA cycle into the daily working of your unit will enable you to anticipate problems at a general level and develop solutions before specific incidents occur. If an incident does occur, you will have a process in place to handle the disruption, keeping chaos and disorganization to a minimum. The PDCA methodology actually saves a busy manager time and aggravation and provides a form of communication to staff about what is happening on the unit.

For example, each nurse on your unit may be responsible for eight or more patients, and each patient may have prescriptions that vary in type of medication, dose, route and time of administration, and frequency of administration. If there is a problem in the delivery of medication, say the Pharmacy didn't send the correct medication or there was a delay in the delivery, the process is halted while the problem is resolved; and many people suffer—not only the patient and the nurse immediately involved, but all that nurse's other patients as well.

As a manager, you want to avoid that kind of disruption of service. If you can anticipate problems and have a plan in place for the delivery of medication, you will have preempted many potential problems. That is good management. Using data collected to monitor the process, you will be able to maintain a seamless and reliable delivery of services. If the PDCA cycle is embedded into the daily functioning of the unit, it will become a normal routine, a way of thinking about care delivery, and it will take very little time.

Plan

The Plan portion is the thinking stage, the analysis stage where you examine your services and anticipate improvements. Begin by analyzing why things are the way they are now. When you study the processes you have, you can discover any obvious flaws that should be improved. This requires information, evaluating internal and external data and the environment of care. Use the tools described in Chapter Five to foster your analysis, especially the cause-and-effect diagram, process flow chart, control charts, graphs, and tables, plus whatever else you think most appropriate.

Consider whether procedures are in place because they were well designed and working effectively, or simply because they evolved over time and no one has thought to evaluate them. Ask yourself if you see any improvements that would make the delivery of care more efficient, of a higher quality, or more cost-effective. Talk to your staff.

Since the Plan phase of the improvement process is a rational and deliberate method to analyze your service for improvement, you (as always) have to think about your customers, the people who benefit from your service. What are their expectations, and are you delivering service to their satisfaction? How do the anticipated improvements interact with the hospital's mission and vision, and leadership's expectations of your services? How would the improvements affect the care on other services? You don't deliver care in a vacuum or function independently of other services, so you need to ensure that your improvement efforts can be coordinated with other departments for the benefit of the whole. What disciplines or staff would ideally be involved in developing these improved processes, and what resources would be necessary?

Your wish list of improvements can be general or specific. For example, if you want to improve the patient flow in and out of your unit, you might have several suggestions for improvement, such as radiological findings reported to the ordering physician within thirty minutes, or beds ready for the next patient within fifteen minutes of the previous patient's discharge. You can gather information from your staff about bottlenecks in patient flow, and when you have compiled a group of factors, the prioritization matrix discussed in Chapter Three can help you determine which issue is most pressing.

With your objectives clearly defined, you improve communication to your staff and together you can develop measures to evaluate your care. It is possible that upon examination and analysis you will discover that the process you are investigating is in fact working smoothly, and the problem that you identified is located in another, perhaps peripheral, process. That is useful information. Or you might discover that the process you are examining is so flawed and full of land mines that it hardly pays to start patching it up. You may determine that a fresh start, an entirely new process, would be better. The Plan stage is where you determine your baseline, identify your goals, develop a team of stakeholders, define appropriate indicators, and outline what best practice would be. Using the PDCA methodology, you and your staff work together, not to find someone to blame for errors, but to look, see, think, discuss, formulate hypotheses and assumptions—and plan, plan, plan.

Do

After you identify opportunities for improvement, you can start Doing—implementing the improvements. You will need to develop indicators with carefully defined numerators and denominators, and to train staff in data collection and analysis techniques. Your data will help you measure where you are at the outset of the improvement effort, that is, establish your baseline, and later, as you continue to collect it over time, data will inform you whether or not your interventions have been effective in achieving your objectives. Once you know your baseline, you may want to determine benchmarks for the process you are hoping to improve, either externally from other institutions or by developing your own internal benchmark.

You need to carefully define accountability during this stage as well: Who is responsible for making the planned changes? How will the new process be monitored? By whom? How often will data be collected? Who will do the analysis? And how will the results of the implementation efforts be communicated? You want to carefully design the implementation stage so as to minimize errors. Planning helps control random mistakes.

Often it makes sense to first test a planned intervention or improvement on a small scale, in the form of a pilot study, and measure its impact. A pilot enables you to evaluate your efforts for design flaws or process problems. It makes practical sense to trial your changes in a limited and controlled environment before rolling them out full force. For example, if you implement a new process for changing the bed linens, you need data to assess if that process is working well and if it is having the desired impact of quick bed turnover and improved patient flow. Test your process for at least three months to gauge its effectiveness.

Check

During the Check phase, you carefully review and analyze the data you have been gathering to ensure that you have the results that your improvement effort anticipated and analyze whether or not your intervention has actually succeeded in making the improvement you expected. Review your indicators and your data collection process for adequacy and effectiveness. The Check phase is where you consider the consistency of your outcomes and the stability of your processes. Control charts are useful here.

The analysis should address the level of success of your interventions. Compare the data you have collected with the baseline established at the outset and determine if the results are what you anticipated, and if not, why not. As you analyze, you continue measuring. If refinements are necessary, either in the improvements you have initiated or in the process, you return to the Do phase and then recheck the results.

For example, if a falls education program was implemented, you need data to prove that it was useful. Was it attended? Were there any evaluative measures to ensure that the information was learned? Was it effective in reducing falls? Or if your analysis uncovered that poor hand-washing procedures were influencing a rising infection rate, what measurements can you use to show increased awareness of preventing infection? When you present data to the caregivers to report on the relationship between hand washing and infection, you can reinforce proper procedures. You can also use data to provide staff on the unit with feedback about the success of policies or improvements.

Habits are very difficult to break, especially habits of behavior. Even when nurses assume a watchdog stance in the ICU regarding hand washing and remind physicians to change gloves and clean their hands, their efforts are often not effective. More effective is illustrating the current infection rate with monthly data. Caregivers become uncomfortable when confronted with numbers that prove that their care may be inadequate. Then they are more likely to change a poor practice.

Act

If, in fact, measurements reveal that you have the outcomes you desired—reduced falls, decreased infection rates, lower LOS, shorter bed turnover time, fewer medication errors, improved patient satisfaction, more complete documentation, and so on—you need to Act, that is, to introduce the improvements into the organization on a broader scale. You do this by communicating the performance improvement initiative and results through the appropriate channels.

In any institution or system, the results of improvement efforts should be shared. If the efforts have proved successful, the organization can establish the changes as a best practice to be adopted by other departments or services. If the effort has not been successful, that information is also useful. Knowing that implementing new processes or procedures or initiating certain changes do not result in improved outcomes and communicating this information across departments can save the expenditure of resources, time, and staff involved with fruitless pursuits.

Most often, improvements are replicable across services. An initiative to improve documentation of a specific procedure on one unit, for example, may easily be adapted to another. However, if the intervention is successful but is not suitable for another unit because of differences in patient population, scope of care, or culture, that is valuable knowledge as well. In that case, you reapply the PDCA cycle, looking for refinements that would fit with the particular needs of the new situation. Another word of caution: just because an improvement effort was successful in a pilot study, that doesn't mean it will necessarily succeed when extended throughout the organization. The constant cyclic quality of the PDCA process prevents your improvement team from relaxing on their laurels.

TEAMWORK

Speaking of the improvement team, its composition is critical to the success of your efforts. Enlisting the support of the experts and the frontline workers in implementing new processes promotes success. You want as many individuals as possible to participate in the improvement initiative because a lone champion of a new process or procedure will not have much of an impact on changing behavior. The greater the buy-in of the members of your team, and the more invested they are in the improvement effort, the easier it will be to institute change because there will be many advocates for the new process. Since you don't operate independently of the other services in the hospital, it is best to enlist team members from various relevant departments. They will not only bring their own expertise to the table, they will also communicate the improvement effort back to their service or department. As manager, and the leader of the improvement effort, you need to keep the team focused on the goal—improving the health status of patients.

As the initiative proceeds, you may want to either refine the group or develop subgroups to target certain specific areas. As manager, you may also have to deal with internal pressures from members of your staff who may create obstacles in taking a new look at the delivery of care, or who may want to be part of the team, or not want to be, or who have an emotional investment in retaining the status quo. A good manager has to attend to the psychological and emotional condition of the staff in determining the makeup of the performance improvement group.

USING THE PDCA

The PDCA cycle is exploratory in nature, as it is a methodology used to investigate and resolve a problem or identify room for improvement in existing processes. Analytic and statistical tools as well as data collection techniques ensure that decisions are based on objective information. Assessing and improving care is not an easy task—and almost impossible to do effectively in isolation. By sharing information and by working in teams to analyze performance—using the PDCA cycle—you can allow information from your unit to contribute to formulating improvements throughout the organization, avoiding redundancies, and developing greater efficiencies by reducing the unnecessary use of resources.

In return, working with the process of the PDCA cycle will be of direct benefit to you because you will understand how your work influences patient care on other units and in other services. If you don't understand how you fit into the bigger picture, when you are asked to make changes in care procedures, you might not really be able to see why you should make any change at all. The following sections describe two performance improvement initiatives—one targeting a specific sentinel event, the other a large ongoing process—to help you see how interconnections among departments work in practice and how a change in one department can influence the workings of the entire organization.

Sentinel Events

Regulatory bodies require that adverse and sentinel events be analyzed for root causes and corrective actions developed to reduce or eliminate the causes of the crisis. The PDCA cycle works well for both analysis and improvement. For example, wrong site surgery is a sentinel event that requires immediate rectification. But why and how does it occur? How often? Under what circumstances? What safety nets can be built into the process to avoid this problem? Since surgery involves so many disciplines and individuals, and is of such high risk to the patient, any initiative to eliminate wrong site surgery must be instituted at the top leadership level.

When our Board of Trustees and administrative leadership prioritized wrong site surgery for a systemwide improvement effort, the Quality Management Department took the lead, and, after conducting a literature search and reviewing the Joint Commission's Sentinel Event Alerts on the subject, began, with a team of experts from across the system who are involved in surgery, to formulate goals for an improvement plan. The objective of the improvement effort was to ensure a safe surgical environment across our eighteen hospitals for the almost 48,000 inpatients and for the 116,000 ambulatory surgery patients who are treated annually in our system.

After interviewing the professional staff involved in surgery and gathering lessons learned from near misses that illuminated opportunities for improvement, the team determined that the existing operative site verification policy required revision. Once it was revised, an educational component to train relevant staff about the new procedures would be introduced, with ongoing education to influence operating room culture, which tends to be controlled by the surgeon, subject to economic pressure for maximum efficiency, and faced with complex new technology and processes.

To analyze the potential causes of wrong site surgery, the multidisciplinary team developed a cause-and-effect diagram that highlighted the major categories that might be involved in an event: staff, procedural setup, preoperative assessment, and environmental factors (see Figure 6.2).

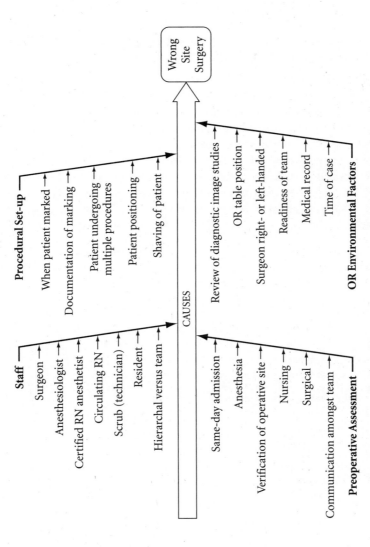

Figure 6.2. Cause-and-Effect Diagram: Factors Influencing Wrong Site Surgery.

This analysis helped us deconstruct the general process into its component parts. Certain issues were illuminated as problems through this analysis and areas for improvement were highlighted. For example, many individuals participate in a surgical procedure, yet the culture is such that the surgeon is considered the undisputed authority. This king-of-the-mountain attitude can affect other members of the surgical team and make them reluctant to suggest corrections. Communication among the OR team was targeted for improvement.

Studying procedures for flaws in the process, the team realized that often a patient's surgical site was marked as required by the policy, but the identification was done after the patient was prepared for surgery, which could result in the marking being responsive to the prep rather than to other, more valid documentation. Although preoperative assessment was expected, the transfer of information was found to be poor, especially for same-day admissions. Environmental factors that had an impact on wrong site surgery included the day's case sequence (the last case proved to be particularly subject to error), the presence or absence of the imaging studies, and how the OR table was posi-

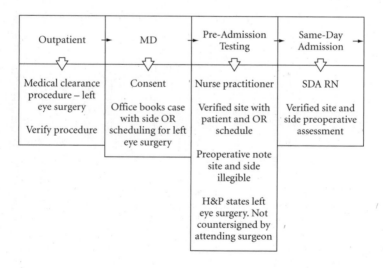

Figure 6.3.   Sequence of Events Chart:
Risk Points for Surgical Procedure.

tioned relative to the surgeon's preference for right- or left-handed work. Managers from Admissions and Radiology and OR technicians, in addition to physicians and nurses, were involved in analyzing the policy.

The cause-and-effect analysis provided general information regarding wrong site surgeries, but to better understand how the process was vulnerable to errors, the team examined a hypothetical event of a wrong site surgery. By outlining the flow of the event, with emphasis on where the risk of incorrect site verification was greatest, the team had another tool to use when considering how best to revise the policy. Figure 6.3 illustrates a horizontal flow chart that defines the sequence of events and the critical stages involved in establishing site verification for a left eye surgery, from the time the surgery is scheduled in the physician's office until the time it is performed—on the patient's right eye.

As the process was analyzed, it became clear how many people and disciplines were involved. In this case, the primary care physician gives medical clearance for left eye surgery. The patient meets with the surgeon,

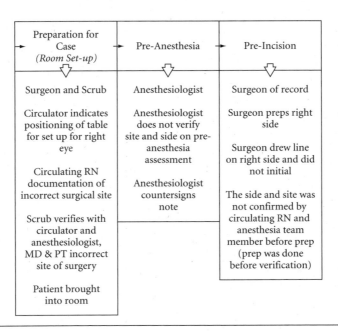

whose office schedules the surgery for the left eye. As required, when the patient enters the hospital for the procedure, the site is verified by the patient and recorded as part of the history and physical (H&P) by the nurse. Further, the plan of care has to be included in the patient's medical record, and be legible as to which eye is involved in the surgery. The attending surgeon is required to sign, and thus to read, the H&P. A series of other steps that are potentially risky to site verification follow, until the surgeon incorrectly preps and then marks the right eye for the procedure.

Doing this specific analysis had the advantage of clearly illustrating problems in the verification process. Presurgical documentation regarding the correct site was illegible; the H&P was unsigned—and perhaps unread as well; the circulating nurse set up the OR for a right eye, making an incorrect assumption; everyone else involved in the surgery responded to the room setup. In addition to a lack of verification of the site from the documentation, there was poor communication among the team; no one questioned or verified the nurse's faulty assumption. In this example, the surgeon prepared the site prior to verification, and marked the site as required, but only after the prep.

After several months of analysis, the operative site verification team developed a revised surgical site verification checklist required for surgery. The new policy mandated that skin prep and drape not be done until after the checklist was completed and signed by the registered nurse and the surgeon. The new policy required that OR documentation verify the surgical site, that the consent form state the site, that there be a documented medical record review by the physician prior to surgery, that patient-specific imaging studies be present in the room, and that there be a pause prior to drape and prep to confirm the correct site verbally and out loud. Only after all that is accomplished is the surgeon allowed to mark the patient. In addition to the new site verification policy and the new checklist, as part of the Do stage of the cycle the team also developed a monitoring form to ensure compliance with the revised protocol.

After the policy had been approved by the medical boards and been in use for six months, the task force reconvened to determine how the new policy was being operationalized. On-site observation and data regarding near misses revealed that the process was still in need of improvement. Therefore, the checklist was revised to include verification both by the patient prior to the administration of anesthetic and by the anesthesiologist prior to the surgery. Another barrier to acceptance of the revised policy came from physicians, who were reluctant to change their tried-and-true (that is, habitual) practices. Targeted education and the endorsement of medical leadership were effective in influencing physicians to comply with the new policy.

Ongoing data collection determined that the revised policy was successful. Studying the charts of surgery conducted over a one-year period, the team collected data on seven critical points, as shown in Figure 6.4.

Data analysis revealed that documentation of the new policy was complied with between 95 percent and 99 percent of the time by the nurse, surgeon, and anesthesiologist. Other data also revealed a reduction in near-miss wrong site incidents.

Results of the data collection were communicated throughout the system. Quality Management staff educated physicians and nurses about the new procedure and about the documentation regarding compliance with the new procedure. In our system, performance data get communicated throughout the organization through the Quality Management committee structure, which transfers information from the unit to the hospital performance improvement coordinating group and then to a system level committee comprising clinical, administrative, and quality leadership and the members of the Board of Trustees. Continuous monitoring reveals that the process is working well. It was determined that the policy be expanded to encompass other procedures such as interventional radiology and not be limited exclusively to those procedures performed in the operating room.

Process Improvements

Another example of how a PDCA intended to improve performance has an impact on many different services involved an investigation into one community hospital's LOS. Administrative data revealed that the LOS at this hospital was high and that the hospital was losing money because insurance companies would pay only for the predetermined LOS for specific diagnoses. A PDCA to address these inefficiencies began with extensive analysis of the situation.

Administrative and medical staff at this community hospital believed that the reason their LOS was so high was because their patients were sicker, older, and had more comorbidities than elsewhere in the system. A team headed by Quality Management, with membership from the hospital's medical, nursing, and administrative staff, analyzed the patient population according to the case mix index (CMI), which is a severity rating of patient illness.

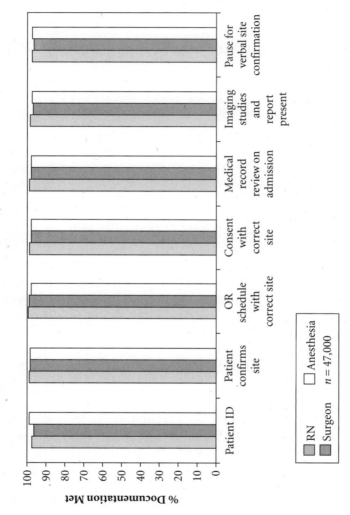

Figure 6.4. Bar Graph: Documented Operative Site Verification.

The resulting data revealed no difference between the severity of illness at this hospital and at others in the system. Figure 6.5 graphs the excess days (right Y-axis) that were being denied reimbursement by the insurance carriers and the CMI (left Y-axis) of seven hospitals (X-axis), showing that this hospital, J, had an unusually large number of excess days for a patient population similar to the others.

To address the problem the team required more information than simply that the LOS was high and the CMI was average. Their data allowed them to go on a fishing expedition and spread a wide net to see if information could be acquired that would pinpoint where the process was breaking down. Until you know what is broken, you don't know what to repair. The team drilled down through the data to see if any particular problem was a major factor. Analysis was made at the unit level, to reveal if a particular unit was responsible for the high LOS, and by diagnosis, to determine if a particular course of illness was causing the problem. LOS was also analyzed according to service, payor, physician, and discharge disposition. No specific problem was identified. Staffing was determined to be adequate.

The next step in the analysis was to do a medical record review of patients and a site visit to get a clearer picture of what was affecting the flow of patients. The medical record review revealed that the plan of care was not clearly communicated, nor was there any evidence that it was addressed by a multidisciplinary team. Communication was poor among the caregivers. Nursing wrote progress notes on a separate paper rather than in the main section of the chart. There were no multidisciplinary rounds. All the disciplines involved in patient care— physicians, nursing, physical therapy, social work, utilization staff— were working independently, in silos, not talking to each other about the patient's care.

For example, a patient with a fractured hip was not getting timely nursing help to ambulate; Physical Therapy consults were delayed; Social Work was not called in to assess rehab needs. Nor was the discharge planner evaluating the type of rehab that would be required. Nutrition was not consulted about particular dietary concerns. Care was fragmented and disorganized. All this has an impact on LOS. Examination of the medical record further revealed that many patients were discharged to nursing homes, a situation that requires Social Work staff to instigate procedures early on in the patient's hospital stay. Further, no one was compiling a census detailing patient information with expected LOS. In other words, analysis revealed that the LOS problem was the result of multiple factors that contributed to a

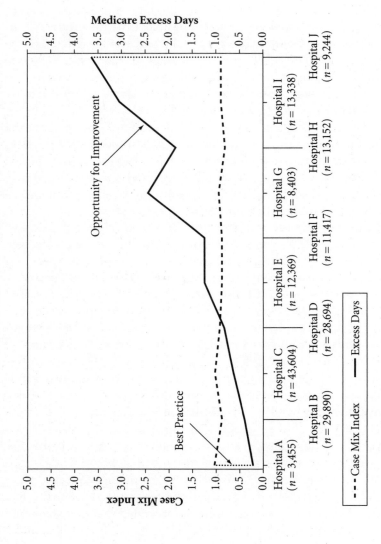

Figure 6.5.   Line Graph: Case Mix Index and Medicare Excess Days, 2002.

disorganized process of patient management and not the severity of illness or other clinical factors.

The team consulted with Information Services (IS) to create a daily census report that included admission date, diagnosis, and anticipated LOS for every patient on the unit, based on the CMS data. The report helped nurse managers, nurses, and Utilization Management staff to prioritize discharge planning based on the patients' characteristics and acuity of illness. High-risk screening criteria were implemented for patients whose needs indicated that they required early screening for postdischarge support.

Multidisciplinary rounds were instituted with a tool for accountability. If one discipline was not present, medical and administrative leadership consulted them for an explanation and Quality Management staff educated them on the importance of participating in daily rounds for improved communication, efficiency of care, and for reducing unwarranted resource consumption. All staff were educated on the use and importance of the multidisciplinary plan of care that was part of the medical record.

Some seemingly simple changes made a great impact. For example, the need for more equipment was revealed through the analysis, especially fax machines to enable floor and unit nurses to quickly communicate with ancillary staff. With the support of the administration, system Quality Management recommended that a new organizational structure be instituted, so that Social Work, Utilization Management, and Quality Management would report to one person in order to enhance communication and accountability regarding the continuity of care.

Standardized criteria were developed to evaluate appropriateness of admission and continued stay, based on severity of illness and intensity of service. Staff were educated regarding the use of the criteria. This change resulted in fewer inappropriate admissions.

A tracking tool was developed for consultations and for reporting of test results. Better monitoring of these services improved timing. Utilization Management made daily reports to the administration about patients' progress through the system. If there was a problem, medical leadership and the administration helped to correct it.

With such a multipronged improvement effort under way, data collection and analysis were crucial to evaluating progress. Data were collected on multidisciplinary rounds, on how the patient's plan of care (clinical guidelines) was used, on discharge disposition, and of course on LOS. Compared to the baseline data, results were dramatic.

LOS decreased significantly. Readmission rates were tracked at the same time, to ensure that patients were not being sent home prematurely. Data revealed that patients were not returning as a result of decreased LOS. Patient satisfaction data improved. Monitoring remains continuous, so that staff can be alerted to any issue that derails the improved process.

This elaborate improvement effort was communicated through the hospital quality structure, in departmental meetings, and through the different service performance improvement groups. The success of the improvement plan was evident, and the impressive results were showcased at these various forums. Accountability was improved, as was multidisciplinary communication. In fact, the hospital underwent a culture change with this initiative. Gone were the independent silos—physicians were now discussing plans of care with nurses, and nurses were communicating to the ancillary staff.

Nursing expressed pleasure at having colleagues available for communication regarding patient services. Patients were pleased not to be kept in the hospital waiting for discharge arrangements to be made. The administration was pleased because hospital income was improving. Physicians felt the improvements because more services were available without delays, and due to improved efficiency, patient complications such as infection were reduced.

This improvement effort took six months to plan, and almost a year to enact. Checking is constant.

Improvements

These two examples show how the PDCA can be used for a single targeted problem and for addressing a general need to improve services throughout the hospital. In each case, many departments and services were involved, as were many managers. Decisions were based on data, and improvements were measured for effectiveness.

The great advantage of the PDCA over other methods of improving processes is that it takes the entire process into account. Therefore the ramifications of the improvements spread throughout various services. And, as we suggested earlier, using a PDCA encourages a culture of multidisciplinary communication and patient-centered improvement efforts. Everyone sees the advantage, both personal and to the patient, of not working in isolation, of planning, of data, of communicating, and of accountability to the success of the process.

SUMMARY

Performance improvement involves the following steps:

- Plan for improvement through extensive data analysis.
- Use a deliberate methodology, such as the PDCA cycle, founded on common sense, data analysis, and education.
- Build an awareness of the interdependence among services and disciplines.
- Change ingrained habits and behaviors.
- Set up ongoing monitoring of services through data and databases.
- Develop a culture where near misses are identified and analyzed to prevent small errors from becoming tragedies.
- Make a coordinated effort among departments and services.
- Consider the resources that need to be spent on the effort.
- Communicate performance improvement objectives to staff.
- Establish accountability for the improvements that are implemented.
- Enroll dedicated champions to educate others about the improvement effort.

It offers the following advantages:

- It helps resolve problems and improve existing processes, and promotes proactive anticipation of risks to patient safety.
- It preempts problems so as to avoid disruption of vital services.
- It makes it easier to respond to the expectations of patients, the organization, and the manager.

Things to Think About

- Data show that your unit has a longer bed turnover time than other units in the hospital. Using the PDCA methodology, outline your performance improvement effort and list the quality tools you would use.
- One of the problems you have to overcome is that your staff thinks this is all a waste of time. How would you convince them otherwise?

CHAPTER SEVEN

Working with Guidelines

I f there are forty patients on your unit, then you probably have forty different histories to understand and forty unique and individualized plans of care to oversee—that is, if all your patients even have an identifiable and articulated plan of care. Each of your patients has a unique physical condition and history along with specific cognitive and psychosocial issues, and will experience treatment in a personal way and recover at an individual pace. The patients you are responsible for are all at different stages of illness, treatment, and recovery. If you don't have an organized process to help you manage your patients, the illness (or the forty illnesses) may begin to control you! You want a process to help *you* control and even predict the clinical situation.

COORDINATING CARE

Moreover, it is not unusual in today's health care environment for each of a unit's patients to be seen by a number of doctors and ancillary professionals. Often, no single physician coordinates a patient's care throughout the hospital stay or communicates the relevant details to the nursing staff as the patient moves through the continuum of care.

For example, patients with congestive heart failure (CHF) may need to be evaluated by several specialists: from Medicine, Nursing, and Pharmacy, and by a cardiologist among other consultants. Each patient will probably require technical tests like EKGs or X-rays, which means that technicians and radiologists will be involved as well. Patients with CHF often need to be seen by Respiratory Therapy and Nutrition. Or the orthopedic patient may, in addition to the orthopedist, require evaluation from an internist to address susceptibility to blood clots, be closely monitored for skin injuries (Nursing), and need physical therapy, nutritional consults, social work involvement, pain management, and home care services. Who coordinates all these services, and how?

Each one of the physicians and other professionals involved with your forty patients may have a different style of interacting with you and with information. And each one probably leaves orders for the care of each particular patient with varying degrees of communicative skill and legibility. If your job is to manage it all, how can you do it without simply reacting on the spur of the moment, making decisions under pressure, hoping for the best, running around like a chicken without a head, or pulling your hair out? You don't need to buy new or more complex technology to manage your patients' care, but you do need a method—a process—to help you organize what has to be done, a process that satisfies the patient, the physician, yourself, your staff, and your supervisor. You need guidelines.

Who's in Charge?

Without coordinated care at the bedside, the patient and the organization are vulnerable both to inadequate care and to financial problems. Administrators typically attempt to resolve the negative impact of poor organization by reengineering the process and encouraging efficiency. However, efficiency alone does not necessarily promote quality care.

If a patient is discharged quickly, LOS might be reduced (efficiency), but if that patient is readmitted within a short period of time, the first admission must be reevaluated to identify any gaps in the original treatment. This reworking of the case is highly inefficient and uses resources that may be costly. In addition, insurance companies frequently won't pay for a second admission that is required not because the first admission was ineffective but because it was incomplete. Generally these problems result from poor communication among the caregivers.

Imagine the following scenario:

An eighty-four-year-old woman, Mrs. P., entered the hospital to undergo cardiac surgery to replace a leaky aortic valve. The surgery was successful. However, because her postoperative care did not follow standard procedures, she developed a secondary illness that became acute. Instead of being a recovering cardiac surgery patient, Mrs. P. was then suffering from a sternal wound infection and required medical attention and a host of ancillary services. The transfer of the case from a surgical to a medical unit did not take place in a timely way, and Mrs. P. developed a painful skin ulcer. Her condition deteriorated to the extent that she required ICU care and several consultations. In the ICU, she became disoriented and delusional.

Prior to surgery, Mrs. P. and her family had determined that she did not want any heroic measures performed, and a DNR order was completed and recorded in her chart. Nonetheless, against the family's wishes, she received a blood transfusion with blood that was not matched to hers and to which she had a severe adverse reaction. Since her condition was going from bad to worse and it appeared that her care was not being managed or coordinated by either an M.D. or an R.N., the family made an official complaint about her care to which the unit manager had to respond, explaining what happened and why it happened. Further, the manager's manager expected that the response would also outline corrective actions to prevent a similar experience.

You never want to be any of the managers involved in this kind of situation—not the recovery room, the ICU, the blood bank, the medical unit, or any of the ancillary services called in for consultation. Mrs. P. exemplifies a patient whose care was random and idiosyncratic and where normal and expected routines were disrupted. If a process had been established and followed in each of the services Mrs. P. required, this scenario could not have happened. Had there been guidelines or norms for standard care during Mrs. P's progress throughout the organization—postoperatively, for skin integrity, in the ICU, and with regard to the ethical issues surrounding extraordinary interventions—the relevant managers would have been alerted immediately that there had been some deviation from the standard delivery of care.

An Organized Plan of Care

Guidelines describe the standard of care for specific diseases or processes. They help in the management of patient care, identifying staff responsibilities and required unit resources by providing a kind of road map for the delivery of services and of expected treatment. What is especially challenging to the manager is to identify problems and issues while care is ongoing, and to coordinate services so that problems can be anticipated and thus minimized. A guideline provides for an organized plan of care because it is a deliberate and formal tool to coordinate and communicate the needs of each patient with the responsibilities of your service.

Think of the diversity of diagnoses, treatments, age, and comorbid conditions on a medical or surgical unit, all requiring multiple services, different diets, and specific treatment plans and approaches to care depending on the psychosocial condition of the patient. To deal with this enormous complexity of services effectively, the manager needs a tool to reinforce uniformity of care. Uniformity does not mean giving medication or food at certain designated times, but rather having the mindset to approach the clinical problem based on scientific evidence. For example, a guideline for treating chronic asthma might include smoking cessation education for patients. That education is not expected to be offered in identical ways to all patients, but it is expected that the education will be uniformly provided and its value in the treatment of the disease recognized by the caregivers who are responsible for the education.

Guidelines also help managers interact with their own supervisors and managers because they are better able to organize the forty-odd different care plans they are managing and can report on resource allocation in an intelligent and informed way. Further, guidelines assist the manager in focusing attention on the process of care and identifying variation from the normal course of care. They outline information about the key issues involved in different plans of care and about appropriate interventions (what, how often, when, and delivered by whom), as well as delineate the expected outcomes of those interventions. Without a good process, a manager can become disorganized; a lack of organization leads to inefficiency and over- or underutilization of services. With a good process, by contrast, the manager has control over the unit.

Crisis Management

Guidelines also offer invaluable support during a crisis. In a patient crisis, if you have no organization, process, or method to efficiently and effectively deal with the situation, resources such as nurses may be diverted, leaving the other patients on your unit without critical services. During a cardiac arrest, for example, you need a preestablished "code" protocol, a procedure or algorithm where everyone knows their role and responsibilities.

Just as fire drills prepare you for how to behave during a threat to the building, crisis plans prepare you to act quickly and intelligently when it really can be a matter of life or death. You don't want to be deciding the best way to proceed during an emergency or wondering which staff members should respond to the crisis and in what way. When you face an adverse event or outcome, you want preestablished guidelines that detail which interventions to offer, such as what medications at what dosage and in what route. Having a guideline can save valuable time as well because complex care information is readily available to everyone involved. As a manager, you can expect your staff to be familiar with the guidelines so that they can react appropriately in an emergency and maintain patient safety.

Developing Guidelines

Guidelines were originally developed to promote improvements in utilization management, in particular, to decrease length of stay during the postacute phase of hospitalization and to monitor inappropriate admission to ICUs. Criteria for admission and discharge were established, as were criteria for triage in the ED, and for quality care, so that appropriateness of resources, timeliness of the delivery of services, and management of crises could be monitored and controlled.

Many clinical and organizational guidelines have been published in the professional literature. Generally, guidelines target specific conditions—heart failure, sickle-cell disease, or depression—or processes and procedures such as operative site verification, pain management, or bariatric surgery. They describe how to best deliver care to patients with these conditions or undergoing these procedures. Guidelines are most often developed by professional societies such as the American Medical Association (AMA) or the Agency for Health Care Policy and Research (AHCPR), or academic physicians, or even federal agencies (such as JCAHO), based on expert literature in the appropriate field and with consensus of recognized experts.

Hospitals also develop their own guidelines, using published sources as a starting point, so that they can tailor the guidelines to meet the needs of their specific patient populations. To develop guidelines, use the PDCA cycle. Form a team of experts from various services to research and brainstorm the best plan of care for a specific problem (P). Once developed, the guidelines need to be implemented (D) and evaluated over time (C), and then revised so that they are maximally useful and communicated (A).

CLINICAL PATHWAYS

Guidelines that outline key interventions and outcomes along a time line for a specific disease are called *clinical pathways.* They delineate the sequence of expected interventions to be ordered by the physician for a specific disease process such as pneumonia or CHF, or for a clinical procedure such as total hip replacement or cardiac bypass surgery. It is important to stress that clinical pathways depend on physician orders and clinical judgment.

Evidence-based medicine drives the guideline and increases productive communication among the health care team but does not supersede the physician. As medical technology and medical knowledge are constantly changing toward evidence-based science, the clinical guidelines in use have to be updated and revised as well so that patients receive the most current standard of care.

The clinical pathways developed and used by our health system have proven successful in monitoring the quality of clinical care delivered, increasing communication among the multidisciplinary care team, improving patient safety, and reducing LOS. The patient-centered pathway integrates the care delivered by various specialties and departments (see Figure 7.1), and the efficiencies generated by deliberate and appropriate communication are responsive to budget restrictions.

Because each pathway is clinically based, the medical board must approve it before it can be implemented. As guidelines, clinical pathways help reduce variation from the standard of care set by the clinical expertise of the institution. Moreover, variation from the standard can be collected as data that are useful in determining whether or not the standard was met—and if not, why not.

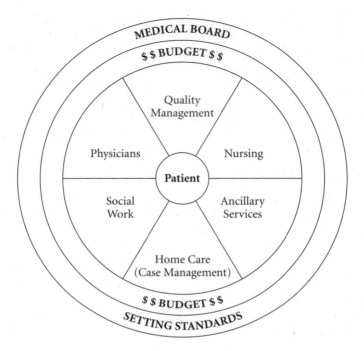

Figure 7.1.   Clinical Pathway Wheel.

Multidisciplinary Teams

The methodology that our health system used to develop these guidelines can serve as a model for others. As with the introduction of any important care process, you need the administrative and clinical leadership to support the effort and to prioritize the project. Once you obtain the commitment to go ahead, multidisciplinary teams then research the literature of a particular disease process to reach consensus regarding the most up-to-date standard of care.

Bringing together a multidisciplinary team not only ensures that the various disciplines involved in an episode of care will have some input, it also increases accountability because everyone on the team acknowledges what is expected. Care delivery is so interdependent that it necessitates that various disciplines coordinate their services. Our clinical pathways delineate how and when that happens, which reinforces communication along the continuum among those who are part of the patient's plan of care.

The advantage of involving the stakeholders in the development of guidelines is that you make use of the local expertise, people who work within the system and can understand its limitations and strengths, and who can serve as champions for new processes and procedures once the guidelines are developed. The more you can involve the stakeholders in the process of developing guidelines, the more empowered they will be. When they know that their input has made a difference, they will more readily adopt and use the guidelines. Participation leads to ownership.

In our health system, individual clinical pathways are reviewed by the department chair or director of the appropriate service, the Medical Board of the hospital, the nurse executive, and the multidisciplinary Quality Performance Improvement Group. Once a guideline is approved, education regarding its implementation takes place in several forums, including multidisciplinary rounds on the floor at the patient's bedside, in-service training, teleconferences, and train-the-trainer programs. The clinical pathways are monitored on an ongoing basis for effectiveness and revised when necessary.

Managing Expectations

The clinical pathway is essentially a cause-and-effect grid that identifies the expected treatment and the expected patient outcome for a specific diagnosis within a time frame. It reflects the physician's plan of care and the current standard of practice, and it targets the interdisciplinary team involved with the patient's care. Clinical pathways, then, are used to plan, deliver, monitor, document, report, and review the care given to every individual patient. Each pathway is individualized for a specific patient, based on the physician's admitting diagnosis and the needs of the patient. Individualized treatment plans increase awareness that treatment has to address the patient's conditions and requirements.

The key clinical markers on the different pathways used in the health system were defined through professional society guidelines and the clinical expertise of the interdisciplinary team as the most important interventions and outcomes to be achieved for optimal care. They identify the critical points during a patient's hospital stay and are evaluated by the relevant department, such as Nursing, Utilization Review, Case Management, Social Work, Physical Therapy, Occupational Therapy,

Nutrition, Pharmacy, and Respiratory, as well as the physicians. Using the pathway ensures that all care providers are on the same page regarding treatment.

CREATING ORDER

Coordinating care with clinical guidelines and encouraging communication among the various disciplines and services responsible for treatment is of great assistance to the manager who needs to organize a unit or service in a coherent way and on an intelligent basis. Because you can anticipate treatment—you know that a patient with pneumonia (or any other disease for which you use pathways) needs this medication on this day or that test if certain criteria are met—you have a basis to predict what staff you might need and which other disciplines or services will be called for.

If more than one patient (of your forty or so) requires similar services, such as nutrition consults, you will be able to organize those services for your entire unit rather than on an individual, patient-by-patient basis. Such information and knowledge allows you to function as a more effective and efficient manager. The managers of the other departments will be better able to manage their staff, schedules, and resources as well.

Most important, in our health system, the clinical pathway is a permanent part of the medical record; therefore all the many people who are involved in a patient's care—doctors, nurses, case managers, social workers, nutrition specialists, respiratory therapists, and laboratory, Pharmacy, Radiology, and Environmental personnel, to name a few—are able to look at the medical record and see at a glance exactly what interventions and outcomes have occurred each day. The effective communication of information that results from having the clinical pathway in the medical record cannot be overestimated. Reinforcing multidisciplinary communication makes the manager's job easier; just imagine how difficult it is to be responsible for informing every single caregiver about the work of every other one. Multiplied by forty!

Variation from the Standard

The more standardized the care you deliver, the more control you have over the delivery of that care. Therefore, it is a great advantage to be able to understand and anticipate the treatment of the disease process and to eliminate, as much as possible, any variation. Clinical pathways help you reduce variation because the expectations for the treatment and the outcomes of the treatment are clearly articulated and understood by everyone involved. The guesswork and randomness of the care processes are reduced.

Each of the 170 pathways currently in use across our health system has five essential parts: a predetermined time frame for the hospitalization, based on CMS or system benchmarks; an up-to-date, evidence-based clinical pathway developed by multidisciplinary consensus; key clinical interventions and outcomes; a list of daily problems with intermediate and discharge outcomes; and a variance analysis record that is removed from the patient's medical record upon discharge.

Any deviation from the standard of care that may influence the quality of care or the patient's outcomes, alter the expected discharge date, or have an impact on the costs of the hospitalization is collected as variance data. Variance data can track interventions and outcomes from the individual caregiver level to the unit level, the hospital, and the system. In our health system, a scannable variance form is completed by the primary registered nurse and sent to the Quality Management Department for analysis. These reports are aggregated and sorted by source of variance, by patient and family, discipline, or practitioner. Therefore, on an ongoing basis, areas of care that need to be better managed can be monitored, and immediate improvements can be instituted if we discover some hole in the fabric of care delivery. Using variance data, general trends in the effectiveness of interventions and outcomes can be aggregated over time for a specific patient community.

For example, if data reveal that in one hospital (or on one unit), blood cultures were taken according to the recommended treatment guideline in only 70 percent of our pneumonia patient population, we have to ask what caused the other 30 percent of our patients not to have this standard intervention. Is this a failure of staff education, or a process problem (the lab got backed up and didn't deliver test results in a timely way, perhaps), or a documentation issue where staff is not filling in the pathway variance form? Once a problem is identified, education and improvements can be implemented—for the hospital or the service, or drilled down to an individual caregiver level. It is also possible that variance data will lead to the conclusion that the pathway itself is not effective and needs to be revised.

Monitoring Variation

Monitoring variation from the expected process alerts a manager to special issues or problems. In other words, the clinical pathways offer you a tool with which to maintain ongoing (concurrent) monitoring of the care on your service and the results to the patient of that care. Since individual nurses treat individual patients, analyzing variance data enables managers and department heads to have access to information about that care. For example, if your variance data indicate that a specific medication was not administered on a certain day, you investigate the reason why. Perhaps the medication was not given in a timely way because the patient has another condition that contraindicates that medication, or perhaps the order for the medication was not written or received, or it was received but it was the wrong dosage and had to be returned to the pharmacy. Information is the most valuable asset for good management and should be filtered to the caregivers at the bedside and to the support staff.

Clinical pathways also inform you about resource expectations, appropriate utilization of services, and lengths of stay typical for specific disease processes. If the key interventions are met, and the outcomes for each day are achieved, the nurse manager of a unit, the utilization manager, the social worker, and others can anticipate when the patient will be discharged, and act accordingly.

For example, the NS-LIJHS clinical pathway for pneumonia lists key treatment options organized by day of hospitalization, as shown in Figure 7.2. On Day 1, a pneumonia patient is expected to have a chest X-ray, blood cultures, a screening for influenza and pneumococcal vaccines, and intravenous (IV) antibiotics administered within four hours of arriving at the hospital. On Day 3, the team is to consider switching from IV antibiotics to oral antibiotics if all outcomes criteria regarding switch readiness are met. In accordance with CMS guidelines, if these outcomes are met, by Day 4 the patient should be switched, and discharged the following day (Day 5).

If you know that the usual LOS for a pneumonia patient is five days, and your concurrently reviewed variance data reveal some variation in the expected interventions or outcomes, you can anticipate that the patient will not be discharged on time and you can investigate the reason. The unit manager and other professional staff can manage the unit's resources more effectively because patient information regarding treatment, outcomes, and LOS is current.

Met	Unmet		Community-Acquired Pneumonia Interventions
✓		Day 1	Chest X-ray
✓			Blood cultures
✓			Screened for influenza vaccine
✓			Screened for pneumococcal vaccine
✓			IV antibiotics within 4 hours of arrival
✓		Day 3	Consider switch to oral antibiotics
✓		Day 4	Smoking cessation education
✓		Day 5	Consider administration of influenza vaccine
✓			Consider administration of pneumococcal vaccine
✓			Discharge

Figure 7.2.   Key Interventions Chart.

Analyzing Variance

Variance analysis supplies useful information about the interventions and outcomes delivered across the health system. For example, the expected outcomes for each patient with community-acquired pneumonia (CAP) (see Figure 7.3) are tracked by day and detail clinical goals. Variance data show how well the plan of care is being followed and how often and why patients are not meeting the pathway goals.

By tracking the aggregated data regarding the percentage of outcomes that were met for CAP patients over a one-year period (see Figure 7.4), the health system was alerted to the fact that discharge instructions were not being delivered effectively. Therefore, improvement efforts could be targeted toward a better process and care improved for this group of patients.

Aggregating data also reveals successes in treatment. For example, when the outcomes of patients with CHF who were treated on clinical pathways were compared with another group of similar patients who weren't, data showed that the patients on pathways had a greater record of nutrition consultations and timely medication delivery than the comparison group. Consequently those patients had less weight gain and were more compliant with dietary restrictions and medication administration. The patients on pathways got better faster and were able to leave the hospital on time with fewer complications.

Met	Unmet		Community-Acquired Pneumonia Outcomes
✓		Day 1	Oxygenation assessment (*ABG or pulse oximetry*) within 24 hours of arrival
✓		Day 2	Exhibits decreased respiratory effort
✓		Day 3	Patient is efebrile
✓			Patient can take oral medication
✓			RR < 24
	✓		Pulse oximetry > 90 or pO$_2$ > 60 mm
✓			Patient pulse < 100
✓			Baseline mental status
	✓		Patient safety increases activity level
	✓	Day 5	Patient verbalizes discharge instructions (*signs and symptoms of complication to report to MD, understanding of vaccines*)

Figure 7.3.   Individual Outcomes Chart.

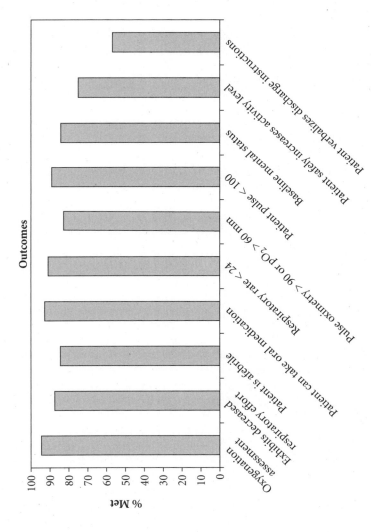

Figure 7.4. Variance Analysis: Community-Acquired Pneumonia, 2002.

Patient safety issues, such as falls prevention, skin care, and pain management are incorporated directly into the different pathways to maintain awareness of these important issues. If not properly managed, these safety issues can prolong a normal LOS. The Utilization Management coordinator or nurse manager can use the pathway to focus the attention of the multidisciplinary team conducting patient care rounds on any variation from the norm. Then the team can evaluate issues identified as having an impact on the LOS or quality of care as well as the discharge planning process for each patient. More information means more control, and more control leads to better management.

Retrospective review of variance data also helps identify potential managed care problems and is invaluable in negotiating and maintaining managed care contracts because payors realize that the organization has a process in place to deliver the most up-to-date standard of care, as well as a mechanism to identify patterns and trends on an ongoing basis. In other words, mistakes or fragmented care that might result in a longer LOS and other issues of concern to payors can be identified through the variance data and corrected quickly. It is crucial to report information from the variance data back to the caregivers (if the care was met or not) so that managers can supervise improvement efforts and monitor and allocate resources.

GETTING EVERYONE ON BOARD

To sum up: clinical pathways help increase communication among caregivers and provide information about the standard of care delivered (or not) to each patient, appropriate to a specific disease process. Implementation of clinical pathways allows the unit manager or department supervisor to create efficiencies of resource consumption and utilization. The pathways tell a story about what should happen, based on the cumulative and aggregated experience of experts. Being incorporated into the chart, they become a permanent part of the medical record, a resource for both retrospective and concurrent analysis of care. In addition to these powerful reasons for using clinical pathways, regulatory agencies like the JCAHO and the Institute of Medicine now recommend that guidelines be used to reduce the gap between practice and the expected and recommended outcome.

Based on all these advantages, it seems obvious that everyone should be happy to be using guidelines as much as possible. In reality, however, because health care is delivered by human beings, there is a great deal of variation in acceptance of these guidelines.

Physicians

Although the guidelines are developed through consensus, there are always outliers, especially physicians, who don't want to be confined (as they might think) to a preestablished plan of care. They feel that their education, expertise, and subjective experience with treating patients are better barometers of care than any clinical pathway. They want the freedom to do what they want to do when and how they want to do it and not to be constrained by policies that require them to deliver care in what they refer to as "cookie cutter" medicine.

Part of the quality challenge for managers, for whom the advantages of using clinical pathways and collecting variance data are great, is to convince physicians and other caregivers that guidelines are simply that—guidelines. They are not meant to dictate every specific incident in the patient's hospital stay, only to provide the broadest outline of what standard of care should be met. Guidelines in fact are designed to be individualized and to tolerate a great deal of individuality in care.

Data can be used to convince physicians about the advantages of following clinical pathways, especially those developed by expert peers who treat the same patient population as the reluctant physician. Individual physicians do not have access to huge samples of patients or of treatment protocols. They trust their own experience, along with the literature, case conferences, and their judgment. And sometimes they need convincing that they should make changes in their care practices. The question is how to bring evidence to bear that will be convincing.

In our system, for example, Quality Management Department data illustrated that within certain parameters (such as normal enzymes), a cardiac patient could be discharged home and have the required stress test on an outpatient basis rather than as an inpatient. Senior Quality Management personnel went on hospital rounds, pockets bulging with evidence from peer-reviewed journals and studies, to educate physicians about the safety of ordering outpatient stress tests.

Over time, the education, documentation, and peer pressure convinced the physicians that a change in their care plan would be better for the patient, length of stay would be reduced, and there would be efficiencies in care and cost savings as a result of the change. Follow-up data reinforced the success of the change in practice. No adverse events occurred; the patients did just as well. Change was reinforced through constant monitoring, education through the variance data, encouragement, evaluation, and feedback to the physicians.

Guidelines can establish treatment protocols on a proactive basis. Rather than responding to some event with a retrospective analysis of what might have gone wrong with a single patient (such as is done in a mortality and morbidity conference), guidelines can improve care for an entire class of patients. Guidelines and clinical pathways articulate a specific algorithm, a kind of "if this occurs, do that," which can work to the benefit of both patient and physician.

If a plumber discovers that the water pressure is low in a house, the usual response is to look for a leak. The effect (pressure) might be a consequence of a cause (leak). One fact indicates that the other might be possible. But imagine that a doctor has a patient whose hemocrit is low after surgery. The doctor, who has done the procedure numerous times and knows it well, sees various possibilities for the low count, such as medications that might thin the blood or the extra fluids being given.

However, a guideline would indicate that the individual experience of the doctor be influenced by the aggregated expertise of the larger medical community. Given this particular surgery, it might read, if the hemocrit falls below a certain level it may indicate a leak, so reoperate and search for the cause. In other words, taking into account other vital information, the hemocrit level could be considered a risk point in the care of this surgical patient. Physicians involved in resident education find guidelines extremely useful, as do nurses for whom guidelines provide a framework for intervention and a mode of communication with physicians.

Guidelines can actually provide physicians with critical information in the case of an adverse event. Imagine that a patient has had an abdominal surgery and has been doing fine. Suddenly the patient dies, and the shocked doctor has no idea why. The chart does not show anything untoward. What should the doctor tell the family? The cause is not at all obvious.

The unexpected death has to be reported to the DOH; Risk Management has to call the insurance carrier to alert it about a potential malpractice claim. The family refuses an autopsy for religious reasons, so there will be no information coming post mortem. Yet an explanation is in order, not only for the family but so that the institution can learn from the event. It is important to determine how this case was different from or similar to others, and if it was unique in any way.

Quality Management and the clinical staff do a review and compare the care to the guidelines, because guidelines encode up-to-date, evidence-based best practices for this group of patients (the ones that have had this surgery). It is discovered that the care that was delivered was entirely appropriate, that the presurgical and postsurgical proto-cols were followed—that, in fact, best practice was followed through-out every stage of the hospitalization, and expectations were met. The physician, the family, the state, and the hospital know they delivered the best care possible and that the death was caused by something en-tirely idiosyncratic that perhaps was unavoidable.

Nurses

Guidelines are of great benefit to nurses as well. However, nurses may need to be taught that entering data regarding interventions, outcomes, and variance is not meaningless paperwork that someone (the manager, the Quality Management Department) requires of them, when they have so much actual bedside care to provide, but that it is instead a powerful tool that can actually make their patients safer and their jobs easier and more efficient. If the manager realizes that nurses require education re-garding the implementation of clinical pathways, it is the manager's re-sponsibility to ensure that they understand that the pathway makes their job more efficient because it delineates and coordinates the plan of care.

Knowing what needs to be done, at what point in the hospitalization and by which discipline, which tests should be ordered, and what con-sults are appropriate allows the nurse to function with a great deal of information and support. If some element of care or intervention is missing or an unexpected outcome appears, the nurse can intelligently explore what should be the follow-up care. Furthermore, the manager and the nurse can better organize ancillary services for the patient, and be secure that social workers, physical therapists, discharge planners, and others will understand their role in the total plan of care.

Think about a change in shift, or a transfer from another unit, and how frequently crucial information does not get communicated. Or a patient's chart that turns out to be missing a note, and the resultant work to discover what should be done. With a pathway filled out, any-one involved in the patient's care can read what was done and what is about to be done, and also see what wasn't done that should have been done. And react appropriately.

Patients

Our system has instituted a patient-friendly version of a pathway, which is another tool to help managers manage. This document out-lines for the patient, in accessible lay (that is, nonclinical) language, what to expect for the hospital stay. It explains the kinds of tests to anticipate and outlines the reasons for doing them; it also offers information regarding the medications that might be given, the kinds of activities that are or aren't encouraged, the role of nutrition and diet in recovery, the anticipated length of stay, and the discharge plans. We find that by allowing patients to partner in their own care, we improve their outcomes and make them more satisfied with their hospital experience.

Patient-friendly pathways are especially useful because information helps relieve some anxiety, and the less anxious the patient, the better the outcome—anxiety can cause complications that delay treatment. By communicating what to expect, offering some explanation for the treatment, and defining that one event will follow another, we help patients and their families prepare for their hospital experience. When patients and their families understand what is happening and are not in the dark and helpless, everyone involved feels better. And less anxious patients and families make the manager's job easier.

Clinical pathways are particularly useful in the preparation for complex treatment such as surgery. After surgery, patients and their families are better informed about what to expect regarding recuperation. Knowing what is normal is reassuring, and the effort to enlist patient cooperation increases compliance with treatment. For example, education about nutrition improved dramatically for our CHF patients because the clinical pathway identifies dietary education as part of the plan of care. With education, the patients were more compliant with their dietary restrictions and thus had better outcomes.

COORDINATING PROCESSES OF CARE

Thus far we have been discussing the advantages of using clinical guidelines to help managers manage their responsibilities. In addition to clinical pathways, the NS-LIJHS uses process guidelines to help staff coordinate processes of care. These guidelines are developed in the same way as clinical guidelines, using literature, professional expertise, brainstorming, and multidisciplinary committees. By developing and implementing guidelines about processes, managers can educate staff on what is expected of them as they deliver care.

Developing Process Guidelines

For example, the NS-LIJHS developed guidelines for assessing, monitoring, and treating acute care patients at risk for alcohol withdrawal.

Our incident database alerted us to the fact that a patient's primary medical condition sometimes masked underlying behavioral health issues. Many patients were found to be entering the system for medical or surgical problems, or through the ED, who were appropriately assessed for their medical condition but not their underlying alcohol or drug problem. Lack of staff awareness of such problems can result in serious incidents, even suicide.

A multidisciplinary committee of experts from across the system convened to develop guidelines to standardize the identification of medical and surgical patients with alcohol problems. Guidelines were also developed to enhance the medical management of these patients. After months of planning, guidelines that included recommended physician order sets for treatment were developed from national guidelines and from internal expertise. A pathway for alcohol detoxification was incorporated into the primary clinical pathway of every acute care patient who, after screening, was thought to be at risk of withdrawal.

Implementing New Processes

The guideline was approved by the medical boards and instituted. Once approved, a new guideline becomes, effectively, hospital policy. Naturally, before implementation, staff had to be educated about guideline use, which was accomplished through a variety of forums, including teleconferences and grand rounds. The new protocol recommended by the guidelines has resulted in initiating adequate treatment in a more timely way for the patients, who are (now) properly assessed. Relevant consults are ordered. All care personnel know what is expected of them. For a manager, it is very useful to have each person's functional role outlined. Guidelines of this type have the added advantage that if a staff member is not familiar with the protocol, it is immediately available for use.

Another process guideline that the NS-LIJHS has recently developed involves bariatric surgery. The system wanted to ensure that this serious surgery be performed only on patients who met specific criteria and only by surgeons who had appropriate training and experience. Safety includes competency, knowing what to do, and when to do the surgery and how, as well as assessing whether or not the patient is appropriate for the surgery and is able to comply with the nutritional protocols.

Lack of compliance can be dangerous for these patients; it can require further surgery or lead to serious complications. The psychological condition of the patient is thus crucial to success. A multidisciplinary committee met for several months to outline the physical and psychological profile of the potential patient and the requirements that had to be met by the surgeon. Such guidelines promote a high standard of care for patients and ensure that established protocols are used to promote maximum patient safety.

THE BENEFITS OF GUIDELINES

Guidelines are the most effective communication tool for the myriad caregivers involved in a patient's hospital stay, ensuring that the treatment plan is articulated and followed, and that guesswork is avoided. Everyone knows what they are supposed to do, and when, including the patient. Proactively, expectations for the most up-to-date standard of care are set, and variance data record if those expectations have been met, and if not, why not. In this way, guidelines provide an educational tool for the individual physician or nurse, the unit manager, the department, and the hospital.

And using guidelines prompts caretakers to think: Were the vital signs taken on schedule? Were the appropriate tests done and the results delivered in a timely way? Was discharge planning begun on time? Did the consults with Social Work or Home Care occur as expected? Was Nutrition consulted, and pain management adequate? Care delivery can be viewed holistically, rather than each caregiver only focusing on a separate small piece of the care process. For the manager or supervisor, guidelines are a most useful tool—for organization of resources, for maintaining and coordinating order at the bedside and on the unit, for understanding and being able to communicate and supervise the delivery of care among multiple patients.

Guidelines are also effective evaluation tools, which can be of great importance to a manager. They expose which interventions are being met and which aren't, who is complying with the guideline and who isn't. Moreover, nurse managers can educate their staff to see the big picture, to understand specific disease processes in a coherent way. Therefore, a single nurse's experience is enlarged by the experience of the expert community. Results of variance analysis can target opportunities for improvements.

Using guidelines also helps demystify the medical process—for the patients, the nurses, and the physicians. There is an orderly plan of care for all caregivers to refer to. Specific disease processes can be anticipated to take a certain course, with treatment deliberately informed by expert information. Guidelines help mediate between the art and the science of medicine, between less and more experience. And for the manager, especially, following a clinical pathway or a process guideline can bridge the gap between less and more organized and efficient care. For a new manager, in particular, this is a welcome tool.

SUMMARY

Guidelines promote improved coordination of care and better management in the following ways:

- They outline the most up-to-date standard of care for specific diseases and processes.
- They provide a road map for the delivery of services and expected treatment.
- They allow for concurrent review of care.
- They provide information for informed resource allocation.
- They offer an algorithm for appropriate care during a crisis.
- They describe how best to deliver care to patients with specific conditions.
- They define key interventions and outcomes for specific disease processes.
- They increase communication among the health care team.
- They identify critical points of an episode of care.
- They identify variation from the standard of care.
- They incorporate information regarding resource allocation and anticipated length of stay.
- They provide a database for analyzing patterns and trends in patient care.
- They incorporate the aggregated clinical experience and expertise of many professionals regarding optimal care.

- They empower the patient with information about the hospital experience.

- They provide an educational tool for caregivers.

Things to Think About

- Why would you make an effort to convince the physicians you work with to comply with the clinical or process guidelines?

- What information would you use to influence their behavior?

CHAPTER EIGHT

Communication and Accountability

ommunication, accountability, and quality are so integrally related that it is difficult to draw lines where one concept begins and another ends. Unless information is transferred effectively, that is, communicated throughout the organization, quality care is compromised. Unless the individuals involved in the delivery of health care services understand that they are accountable to the patient, the institution, and their colleagues, and that their accountability includes effective and open communication, quality care is diminished.

From the top leadership to the hourly workers, everyone involved in health care should feel responsible not only for the particular service they deliver but for the entire process of care. The activities of one person affect many others because care is so interconnected. Having pride in the organization and pride in one's work goes hand in hand with accountability. You want people to know when you have done a good job; and you want others around you to do their jobs well. To deliver quality care, the organization needs a culture that welcomes effective communication as well as a defined structure that serves as a conduit for carrying that communicated information throughout the institution.

A COMMON GOAL

Communication is not solely about the transfer of factual information; it incorporates the ideal of working together toward a common goal, and finding a medium, whether committee meetings, e-mail, oral directives, or hand gestures, to do so. It is not the particular style of communicating that needs to be shared, only the goal of the communication— to deliver the best quality patient care. If everyone involved in an episode of care focuses on the patient, the value and power of communication is obvious. Hoarding information, or thinking that no one needs to know what you know about handling the patient, is tantamount to withholding care because the patient can be harmed. Sharing information improves care.

Joining Forces

What can you, as the manager or supervisor, do to improve communication among your staff and throughout the organization? Serve as an example. Set up expectations. What you value filters down to your staff.

If your door is open, if you ask questions and listen to the answers, if you allocate responsibility to others, making them accountable for their work, and require them to report (in whatever form) back to you and to other members of the staff, communication will be seen as prized. If you use language to explore issues and problems rather than to cover them up and try and make them disappear, your staff will learn to communicate honestly also.

You can't be effective at your job—the job of managing each patient's environment of care, of ensuring that the nurses share information across shifts, that the physicians and the nurses understand each other, that the patients' and their families' expectations are met, that your staff has the education they need—without excellent communication. It is much more difficult to communicate effectively than to simply ignore, nod, and shut the door, but it is certainly worth doing. Poor communication will require endless hours of work to repair mistakes, handle complaints, or respond to your manager's and your colleagues' requests.

When services are less than optimal, or when a problem arises, it is most productive to open a dialogue about what went wrong. It is usually pointless to blame someone or to start yelling, "Who was responsible for that?!" Blaming is easy, and in fact takes away from the responsibility and accountability for good care. Blaming simply makes the people who get blamed feel bad about themselves. It does not improve the quality of care one bit. Human beings make mistakes, of course, and blame, shame, and reprimands might make managers feel better about their role and responsibility in a problem, but it does not further the goal of delivering good services. So forget about the blame game and work to create an environment where information, even unpleasant or compromising information, is freely shared.

Whose Job Is It Anyway?

Understanding the role of communication and accountability among disciplines and services, so essential to quality patient care, has evolved over time. Just a few years ago, it was still acceptable for different disciplines and services to operate independently, with little overlap or shared accountability for the processes of care. Because physicians and nurses were accountable for patient care, patient care was thought to be exclusively a clinical issue rather than a hospital, organizational, or societal one.

Determining the quality of care was also thought to be the purview of the medical or clinical staff, the specialists who delivered care, and was considered a separate and distinct piece of the organization, not entwined with organizational or administrative issues. Administrators did not regard quality as a force that could be used to improve the organization because the idea that quality care could be monitored, measured, and evaluated was somehow not apparent to them. Administrative responsibility focused on issues of reimbursement, which seemed to have little connection with quality care.

In the case of an adverse event, physicians were accountable primarily to each other through a peer review process, the mortality and morbidity (M&M) conference, which served as a kind of quality control over the delivery of care. The M&M conference works under the assumption that clinical experience and judgment can provide information as to why complications (never mistakes) occur, with more experienced physicians teaching less experienced ones. During the M&M process, physicians review a particular situation, focusing on the physician's actions and not on any other factors (such as the environment or processes) that could have contributed to a poor outcome. Analyzing root causes of poor outcomes is not part of the process, nor is establishing improved protocols so that certain complications or sequelae can be avoided in the future.

Those individuals who were working in quality were working within a quality assurance (QA) model that was primarily limited to ensuring that regulatory requirements be met. QA personnel were not expected to interpret care or to understand care delivery, only to ensure compliance with regulations so that the hospital would be reimbursed by Medicare and Medicaid.

Working within a QA framework, each incident or lack of compliance was considered unique. For example, if a patient's medical record did not include a history and physical report, this was identified as a problem, but not because its absence had any impact on the patient's care or revealed anything about the process of care—only because it was not in compliance with regulations. QA was expected to identify a problem but had no methodology for preventing the same problem from recurring again and again.

Accountability for the delivery of care was very local; managers were responsible for what happened on their unit or service but not for aggregating, analyzing, or making improvements or for interacting with other services. If a medical error occurred, a single individual was deemed responsible and disciplined accordingly. In other words, errors and the response to errors did not have ramifications beyond the single incident. No one in the organization, not the physicians, the administrators, or the quality personnel, was accountable for an organized and deliberate process to deliver quality care and improved patient outcomes.

INTEGRATING QUALITY
THROUGHOUT THE SYSTEM

The NS-LIJHS moved from a QA model of problem identification toward a fully developed and integrated quality management program that involves every layer of the organization, and our experience might be instructive. In large part, the impetus for change came because the administration at a teaching hospital was concerned that the hospital was receiving repeated deficiencies from the JCAHO and because it had no mechanism in place for dealing with denied claims from the local Peer Review Organization (PRO). Understandably, leadership was worried about these regulatory problems and the financial situation and looked to the Quality Assurance Department to help resolve them. Also, at about the same time, the CEO, a remarkably visionary businessman, learned that the length of stay for certain disease processes was significantly less in California (and therefore expenses were lower) than in his institution and came to QA to ask why.

Developing Connections

Quality Assurance staff saw this challenge as an opportunity to make sweeping changes in the hospital culture: introducing data as basic to monitoring care, enhancing accountability, and improving communication. We convinced the CEO that with leadership support and resources to create a database that could be managed by data analysts, we could reduce LOS and save money. It was our idea that by developing comparative databases, measuring performance by disease, and providing ongoing education to the medical staff, we could illuminate opportunities for improvement and reduce variability in the delivery of care, and so improve utilization.

It seemed clear from past experience that examining any phenomenon in isolation would not further the goal of understanding how a problem developed or help us discover an appropriate solution. To analyze the LOS situation, we had to understand the entire process of care—from the ED, the admission process, and the treatment cycle, through discharge planning to posthospital care—as well as examine the personnel involved and the risk points in service delivery. LOS was a global problem for the hospital and not limited to any specific condition or particular physician. It was, we believed, a process problem where delays could occur at any point. By conceptualizing the problem in this way, the focus changed, moving from the QA model of assessing discrete problems to analyzing processes of care in order to improve results, that is, to a quality management framework.

For example, the LOS for a patient who had suffered a stroke could be influenced by the way the patient's acute care phase was managed by the physician and also by many other factors, such as the availability of rehabilitation services, the patient's response to medication, transfer issues from one level of care to the next, family support or the lack of it, the physician's response to discharge, or home care problems involving Social Work.

At that time, Social Work, Utilization Management, Discharge Planning, and Home Care, all involved in LOS, were independent entities, without open and easy channels of communication, and worse, without any reason to communicate. The key players—the patient, the physician, and the nurse—were also out of the loop. No one was looking at the process of moving a patient along the continuum of care; only the last phase of the patient's stay was examined to discover why the patient remained hospitalized.

In addition, in their efforts to reduce LOS, discharge planners were concentrating their energy on the most complex cases because those had the longest LOS. Therefore LOS analysis concentrated almost exclusively on the outliers, a group that made up only about 5 percent of the patient population; vast resources were engaged in an attempt to understand a problem that affected very few patients. The discharge planners believed that if they could make an impact on those cases, reduce the group that had longest lengths of stay, they would then reduce the LOS on the unit.

Focus on the Entire Process

Rather than focusing on those few outliers who were skewing the LOS data, we took an alternative approach and realized that if we found the common denominator linking the majority of the patients and made an impact on them, we would have much greater success than if we analyzed the care of a few special cases. (Remember the bell curve of normal distribution with the majority of cases around the average and a few outliers on the ends.)

Our analysis revealed that the median LOS was high; therefore it was not solely the outliers who were responsible for the LOS. Instead of increasing the staff resources to discharge those 5 percent of the patient population who were staying the longest, we used the PDCA methodology to examine the entire process of care. Our goal was to understand why so many of our patients were hospitalized beyond what the government thought reasonable and would pay for.

We looked at how communication was working throughout the continuum of care, from admission through treatment to discharge, and attempted to discover what (if any) information was being communicated to whom about the patient. Figure 8.1 illustrates the many people and services involved in the three major cycles of an episode of hospitalization.

For care to be efficient, we needed smooth communication within and across these cycles. We followed the process, moving through the cycles and the transitions between cycles to determine how and from

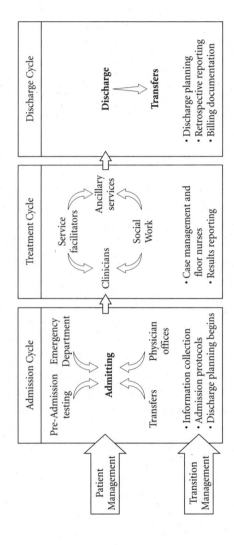

Figure 8.1. Communication Across the Continuum.

where services were provided, who was accountable, and what information was essential to move the patient efficiently through the continuum of care. Without analysis there was no way to ascertain if high LOS was a process problem (about coordination), or involved clinical issues (comorbidities of patients) or some other factor that could be beyond our control, such as the availability of community resources to the patient after discharge.

Redefining the Issue

The concept of reimbursement for utilization has the interesting result of making accountability for patient care somewhat remote from the caregiver and patient. Reimbursement is more a product of administrative and budgetary decisions than it is of bedside care concerns. Our analysis revealed that what drove LOS was external: when reimbursement allowed a prolonged LOS, the LOS was long; when it did not, LOS went down. Patient management by the nurse and the physician were removed from the formula.

However, the concept of payment for services, which seems to be the direction of the future, has another slant, and requires that different questions be asked. For example, what is the payment for? Is it possible to have a positive margin and reduce LOS? Are the number of resources available to the patient too much, too little, or just right? The idea of efficiency focused attention on appropriate utilization of resources and services.

To determine if the LOS for each patient was excessive or appropriate, we needed patient-level data. The quality management staff communicated with physicians and nurses in an effort to become educated about the kind of care that was delivered in different and specialized units, and heard the expected response that because the caregivers were providing high-quality care, the LOS was appropriate. According to the physicians, their patients were sick and required hospital services. Period. End of discussion. The only way we would change their minds, and thus their behavior, was to present comparative data by diagnosis, controlling for demographic factors, hospital size, and comorbid conditions.

Developing databases and a methodology to examine the relationship among variables continued to shape the transformation from QA to Quality Management. But acquiring data was only a first step in changing physician behavior. The medical staff required an explanation as to whether or not the relationship was significant and at what statistical level; these inquiries forced Quality Management to explain the delivery of care by making use of a scientific methodology that was familiar to the physicians.

Show Them the Numbers

Research analysts were hired to design and organize databases for a comparative analysis to be presented at grand rounds and any other communication forum that was available. After comparing our LOS with that of other hospitals in our area according to specific diagnoses and diseases (DRGs), we established benchmarks for appropriate lengths of stay. For example, if a patient with pneumonia or CHF stayed at a neighboring hospital for a day less than at our hospital, we wanted to know why. What made the difference? The process of inquiry and explanation took close to eight months.

We conducted a literature review to ensure the validity of the information we were giving to the physicians and did a comprehensive analysis of the variation from the norm by unit level, floor, and physician for the same DRG. We compared our LOS not only to regionally comparable institutions but went further and compared ourselves to more distant hospitals delivering the same kind of acute care services—city hospitals, tertiary teaching hospitals—as we did. When we found variation in the LOS, we tried to tease apart the reasons for the differences. Some practices clearly prepared patients for timely discharge, such as the switch from IV to oral medication or the provision of IV medication at home with home care supervision. Were these practices available to our patients?

Regulatory agencies also provided data that could be used for benchmarks. The Health Care Finance Administration (HCFA, now CMS) reviewed patient information and care delivery. Each state has a peer review organization (PRO) that monitors the quality of care and conducts utilization reviews for Medicare patients. The PRO provides standards for the number of days deemed appropriate for a specific process, disease, or procedure, after which a patient was expected to be switched to another level of care.

The PRO also helped develop general definitions for acute care and nonacute care. Acute care patients could be identified as having certain symptoms, such as requiring IV medication or having unstable vital signs or certain blood count, sputum cultures, fever, and so on.

Organizations such as the Centers for Disease Control and Prevention (CDC) established other kinds of criteria, such as for defining infection. They also suggested services that should be provided, such as isolation rooms or aggregation of infected patients, to promote prevention and treatment.

Understanding Variability

The Quality Management Department made use of these external guidelines to help define and standardize care. Once it was established that indeed there was variability in LOS per specific disease process, we again needed to ask questions and communicate with the frontline caregivers. Perhaps it was true, as the physicians claimed, that patients in our hospitals were sicker, older, or had more comorbidities than those at other hospitals.

To address these possibilities and to make for a more meaningful comparison, risk-adjusted models were developed to control for variability in clinical symptoms and comorbid conditions. Then we reviewed the nurses' records and the medical charts. We asked about specifics in the delivery of care, looking for commonalities. For example, a stroke patient on Heparin (a blood thinner) could be sent home once switched to another type of medication (Coumadin) that is taken orally. That change in medication, ordered by the physician, served as the spark that initiated the discharge process.

Physicians were not especially pleased to be interviewed by the Quality Management staff about why and when they determined a patient was ready to switch medications. They expected to be fully in control of this clinical decision. But in order to understand the reasons for the switch from IV to oral medication so that we could influence the process and thus the LOS, we needed information, the kind of information about processes that is useful to unit managers who can establish databases to help manage their departments efficiently.

Our interviews uncovered the fact that sometimes the decision to remain on Heparin was not in fact based on clinical reasons. For example, if the laboratory results showed that the patient could be switched from one medication to the other, yet this information didn't reach the nurse or physician in a timely way, the patient would remain in the hospital unnecessarily because of the inefficiencies in the communication processes. Other processes were also affecting LOS. If a patient with any condition was ready to be discharged on a Friday afternoon and Social Work could not be sure that the patient's home was a safe environment (perhaps there were stairs), the patient was kept in the hospital throughout the weekend. As an alternative, patients could be discharged to another, lower level of care, which would care for the patient as needed and still improve LOS. The entire continuum of care had to be considered in the patient experience; such coordination of services takes place on the unit level and is the responsibility of the manager.

Aggregated data showed that most stroke patients had normal blood levels and were ready for the switchover in medication after four or five days. The clinical literature reinforced this time frame as well. But the physicians, each taking care of their own patients, had no access to or awareness of the aggregated information. Quality Management staff showed them the data, collected over a period of time, risk adjusted, and benchmarked against similar hospitals, that proved that most patients were ready for the switch at Day 4, and that delays were occurring for other than clinical reasons. Again, it falls to the manager to establish open communication with physicians so that they can participate in forming a health care team to care for the patient.

Quality Management, using data, was able to prove that communication issues were often responsible for inappropriate resource utilization and high LOS. Each of the many different departments involved in managing the stroke patient was working in independent isolation, and each had an independent objective that was not coordinated in any way with the objectives of the other services. To improve quality and enhance accountability in the delivery of care, it was apparent that barriers needed to be removed from the communication flow and that multidisciplinary teams had to be established so that communication and information among the relevant departments could be linked. We found this to be true not only for stroke patients but generally for many disease processes. Therefore, effective communication among caregivers became a priority for quality management.

Think Globally—Act Locally

The Quality Management Department enlisted the managers to improve communication and accountability. The goal was for leaders of services and departments to think globally about the patient's hospital experience so that they could begin to understand how their service interacted with other units and services throughout the organization.

Changing entrenched behavior, however, is very difficult. To make our case, we went to the units, believing that in this instance a personal appearance would be a more effective communication method than a written document, and educated managers about quality issues, hoping to influence the way they thought about the delivery of care. A seamless delivery of care, from admission to discharge and beyond, requires that the managers each understand their role as part of a whole and know that what occurs on their service has repercussions and an impact beyond their single unit or service.

We began to educate the managers on quality management methodology. For example, we asked the managers and the nurses questions related to general processes of care, such as to articulate the admission criteria for their particular unit, to explain what kind of pain management techniques were being used, or to describe what kind and how many medication reactions occurred weekly on their unit. Understanding how care was delivered on a greater than individual patient level was obviously useful for planning how to achieve daily goals, for the manager as well as the nurse on the floor, but such a framework was a new way of thinking about the delivery of care. We found that these questions provoked interest and even excitement. When managers expect a high level of competency from their staff, the staff responds. Bedside caregivers were expected to know the answers to these kinds of questions and managers were expected to know which of their caregivers could answer such questions and who needed more education.

Most managers realized that Quality Management appreciated the vital role they played within the organization and that the bar was being raised regarding the extent of their information and the quality of the care their service delivered. The more competent and knowledgeable they were, and their staff was, the better their unit would run. Nurses or managers who had wanted to improve the care they delivered were interested in understanding quality management methods, such as the value of indicators, data collection, and analyses. As managers learned the advantage of using data to monitor and improve efficiency, education, communication, and accountability among staff increased. As we eliminated causes of variability and stressed the value of standardization, utilization of resources became more efficient and LOS decreased.

Reaping Rewards

Bringing together the various departments involved in an episode of care improved communication and refined the discharge process. Because caregivers realized that their service was interrelated with others, accountability for efficiency increased as well. The Quality Management staff developed objective criteria for discharge that were applied as early as admission and took pains to explain how each discipline or service fit into the process of moving the patient through the continuum of care. Quality management techniques, such as aggregating data, benchmarking, and using multidisciplinary teams to improve patient care, created clinical accountability for an entire class of patients.

This was a great improvement over the previous system of having a case manager evaluate the situation of each patient separately, one at a time. With aggregated quality data, we could even report success to the hospital administration, which investigated, for example, unplanned readmission. Our data showed that although LOS had been reduced, the unplanned readmission rate did not increase (see Figure 8.2). Thus numbers substantiated our claim that integrating quality into clinical services was productive—for the patient, the organization, the physician, and the regulatory agencies.

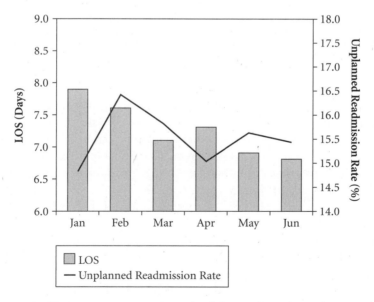

Figure 8.2. Average Length of Stay and Unplanned Readmissions Within Thirty Days, 2003.

Monitoring and Evaluation

An intermediate step between transforming a quality assurance model to a quality management one was the evolution of the role of Quality Department staff in monitoring and evaluating care. This model required that indicators be carefully defined, using numerators and denominators; indicator definitions relied on understanding a class of problems for a specific population. The monitoring and evaluation model, rooted in data, made it possible to define best practices and opportunities for improvement for the hospital, service, and unit.

Quality Management staff especially wanted to know if a problem was a unique, one-time episode or an event that occurred with some frequency. In the latter case, the process needed to be analyzed, understood, and improved. For example, if we saw that x percent of patients in the ICU had nosocomial pneumonia, we could trend this rate over time and see if it decreased. If not, we could analyze what factors could be improved in order to decrease it. What was causing the pneumonia? Perhaps nursing care, or a medication issue, or something as simple as hand washing when moving between patients? Or if the wrong blood was given, rather than blaming the individual who gave the blood, we analyzed the entire process: who ordered the blood, who transcribed the order, who picked up the wrong blood, who transported it, who administered it, where the documentation was along the way, and so on.

Every division in the hospital began to have relevant quality indicators available to measure delivery of service: the ICU collected data on infection, the ED on patients who left without being evaluated. Medical units reported on falls and pressure injuries; the Pharmacy collected information about potential and actual medication errors. Quality indicators were used to quantify care, to interpret it on a level where information could make an impact and improve the delivery of care to the greatest number of people.

Over approximately four years, the monitoring and evaluation function of Quality Management expanded further to include problem solving. Emphasis changed from describing care to improving care. Managers became more adept and comfortable with the idea of quantifying care with numerators and denominators. The ongoing data measures that were being communicated via the multidisciplinary quality performance improvement committees helped managers identify problems and plan for performance improvement.

As the JCAHO required more and more information and an established method for performance improvement, Quality Management adopted the PDCA methodology and the ten-step JCAHO plan for performance improvement. The methodology of PDCA helped to merge problem identification and ongoing measurement with an identified scope of care—defining what type of patient, service, technology was offered—which in turn described what kind of care was being delivered and how effectively it was delivered.

ESTABLISHING A COMMUNICATION INFRASTRUCTURE

As processes became more integrated and efficient, LOS was in fact reduced in the majority of cases, with the concomitant effect of increasing revenue to the institution. Since improved clinical and utilization outcomes were so clearly apparent, administrative leadership and the CEO became champions of quality methodology. However, the Board of Trustees still had reservations. Accountable to the patient and to the community, the trustees wanted to be sure that the patients were happy with the shorter LOS and didn't feel they were being rushed out the door prematurely. The Quality Management response was to collect data to find out.

Patient satisfaction surveys regarding LOS were analyzed. Results revealed that keeping people in the hospital for eight days when they were ready to be discharged after four in no way improved the patient experience. In fact, patients were more satisfied and had fewer complications (such as infections) with a shorter LOS. Quality Management was able to reassure the Board of Trustees and the clinical and administrative leadership that patients were being discharged appropriately because data monitoring such quality indicators as unexpected returns to the OR, unplanned readmission to the hospital within thirty days of initial discharge, or nosocomial infection rates showed no increase.

Forging Relationships

When the CEO and senior leadership saw that administrative goals and those of the Quality Management Department were entirely compatible, they increased their support of the quality management methodology. The CEO began to expect the medical staff to think in a quality management framework and be accountable for the LOS of their patients and justify a longer than expected hospitalization. Most physicians did not want a higher LOS than their peers—especially when the clinical literature and comparative benchmark data supported a shorter one. The role of quality management was to educate the medical and clinical staff to look at aggregated data about the particular disease process, rather than focusing exclusively on an individual patient.

To do this, we made rounds with the chairs of departments and asked physicians to justify why a given patient was still in the hospital, why if the lab results showed someone was ready to be switched to oral medication the IV was still hooked up. Or when we did rounds in the ICU, we asked physicians why their patients were there, without any interventions, simply waiting for a stress test. Integrating quality management data and procedures into the daily working of the unit and maintaining vigilant utilization management increased the managers' leadership role and responsibility to the organization because they were accountable for the activities on their unit.

From the Bedside to the Board

Regulatory agencies require that health care organization board members be accountable for the quality of care delivered in their institutions, but they do not dictate what structure is required or who should participate. When we began the move to a quality management process, Board meetings generally centered on issues of acute care services because they were so pressing. However, the other important dimensions of a hospital also had to be managed, such as the continuum of care after discharge, home care services, ambulatory services, behavioral health, and support services that traditionally are not discussed in medical board meetings, such as environmental services and safety. The communication about quality of care to the governing body typically goes through the medical boards.

The Board of Trustees was extremely interested in understanding the quality issues that the hospitals in the system confronted and wanted to stress the accountability of the medical staff regarding quality. A new high-level committee was formed, the Joint Conference Professional Affairs Committee (JCPAC), to provide physicians, nursing staff, and Board members with a forum for communication. This multidisciplinary quality committee comprised administrative staff, physicians, nurses, and ancillary and quality management specialists; it met monthly to communicate about standardizing care, medical staff credentialing, reducing variation, and ensuring appropriate utilization and reduced LOS.

The Board of Trustees requested a monthly report from the Quality Management Department regarding LOS and its impact on patient care—which meant an analysis of several other quality indicators. Being laypeople rather than clinicians, Board members expected more than numbers on a spreadsheet; they expected an analysis of what those numbers meant in terms of patient care. In time and with education, as Board members became more knowledgeable about quality indicators and understood how integrating quality processes and methodology into clinical services and organizational processes was valuable, they expected more accountability from physicians about quality care and required information directly from them regarding their delivery of services.

If a patient had a long LOS, or a particular physician's patients had a longer LOS than those of other physicians with similar practices, Board members wanted to know why, and more important, what could be done to improve matters—both the care and the LOS. To explain, individuals and disciplines that had previously worked independently were forced to communicate with each other around a common topic (LOS, infection); the most efficient way to do this was to establish multidisciplinary teams to analyze and report out on a topic. These teams became responsible for improving performance and were accountable to the CEO and the JCPAC. The Quality Management Department was able to provide useful data and analyses. The unit managers also saw the advantages of working in a multidisciplinary environment.

As quality topics were discussed in more depth and in broader range, it became apparent that a single committee could not meet its obligation to address the issues and concerns of all the services. Therefore the Board of Trustees' quality committee was separated into other committees with specialized responsibilities, forming, in addition to the JCPAC for acute care and behavioral care, a JCPAC for ambulatory, home care, nursing home and rehabilitation, and safety, which was an outgrowth of security, infection control, and environment of care services. In each of these committees, analytic processes used to understand adverse events, such as root cause analysis and failure mode and effects analysis, were discussed as were important topics such as medication errors and nosocomial infections. The committees shared comparative data to define best practices as well.

A quality committee was established where the chair of each JCPAC would meet quarterly to present its specialized priorities and concerns to the entire group. This group established policy on quality, such as patient safety and patient identification. From the quality committee, topics are presented to the executive committee of the Board of Trustees, where such issues as sentinel events and broader issues on quality such as competency or environmental issues are discussed.

The importance of the quality committee structure is that it gives a voice to the care providers—the physicians, nurses, and ancillary workers—to express their concerns, doubts, and prioritizations in a constructive forum that helps decision makers at the CEO and board level take action in formulating policies and procedures for the health care system.

Building Bridges to Improve Care

With this new mindset of improving care through quality management processes and methods, when one of our institutions was ranked poorly because of a high mortality rate for cardiac surgery, administrative leadership looked to the Quality Management Department to provide analysis of the problem and develop possible solutions. To promote communication among the personnel involved in the care, we established an interdisciplinary performance improvement team.

Integrating the delivery of care for cardiac surgery required a radical switch in mindset for the staff and a culture change in the organization. Just as with the LOS improvement initiative, we needed to use data to influence behavior. When we interviewed the surgeons as to why mortality was so high in cardiac surgery, they responded that their patients were sicker than the average and therefore at higher risk for mortality. Although risk-adjusted data revealed that this was not the case, some physicians were able to convince themselves that since their skill could not be questioned, the published data must be completely incorrect.

Then what was going wrong? The governing body expected an explanation for why the mortality rate was higher than the state's average and suggestions about how to improve. Their challenge to administration and the medical staff forced these groups to take the data seriously and to implement a quality management approach to cardiac services. Everyone involved in the entire continuum of care for the patient admitted for cardiac surgery was interviewed. What was the admission process? What tests and processes were typically administered? What problems occurred? What information was gathered? How was the competency of the caregivers evaluated, and by whom? How were patients prepared for surgery? What was the relationship between postoperative bleeding, infection, and mortality?

Quality Management staff was not surprised to discover that communication was poor. Nurses were making notes that the physicians were not reading, and vice versa, and the cardiologists were not communicating with the cardiac surgeons. Each instance of mortality was analyzed; each event was drilled down to establish the root causes involved. Through this process information emerged that enabled us to define best practices and to develop algorithms for care, such as eliminating aspirin before surgery because it tended to increase bleeding, improving the prescreening process for surgery, and introducing intensivists to supervise postoperative care.

By examining the number of unplanned readmissions through the quality incident reporting system, we discovered that the rate of infection following surgery was high and educated nurses about postoperative infection care. We also enlisted infection control practitioners to help prepare patients for surgery, which we felt would reduce postoperative infection as well. Working together, within a year we had brought the mortality rate down, and within two years, our system was ranked the best (lowest) in cardiac mortality rates. Only quality management methods could have effected such a massive change. With successes like this, we constructed bridges between quality and the medical and nursing communities.

The success of the LOS and cardiac surgery initiatives provided Quality Management with several physician champions who understood the importance of open communication and worked to further the cause of integrating quality management methods into every service and discipline. We made a convincing case that adopting quality management methodology resulted in improved care, greater patient safety, and fewer adverse events.

As the medical staff became convinced that they would be well served by participating in quality improvement efforts, they communicated more information about their cases, enabling us to develop more sophisticated and complete indicators and databases. Being affiliated with a good hospital, that is, a hospital that was recognized for delivering quality care, would be of professional benefit to the physicians as well. They got on board.

IMPROVING PERFORMANCE

LOS reveals a great deal about the quality of care being delivered in a health care organization and locates areas where performance requires improvement. Good care is efficient care, with everyone doing the job they are expected to do and doing it well. If a patient wasn't discharged home because of a delay in preparing the discharge instructions, then a bed was not available to someone who needed it. If the bed wasn't prepared for lack of sheets to put on it because of a holdup at the Laundry or at Housekeeping, a patient could not be moved into it. If no personnel were available for transport, then the patient stayed put.

If a diabetic patient was given an improper diet and complications resulted, or was left immobile for too long and developed a pressure injury, that patient stayed longer in the hospital than would otherwise have been necessary. If an equipment problem or staffing inadequacies meant that a patient fell and required surgery, that patient stayed longer than anticipated. If a patient was discharged too early and had to be readmitted to the hospital, reimbursement would be affected.

Quality meetings for performance improvement came to include Environmental Services, Housekeeping, Nutrition, Infection Control, and Transport as well as the traditional clinical and administrative people. Now, everyone involved in patient care had an opportunity to communicate and to feel responsible for maintaining quality. The quality meeting was chaired by a physician who was charged with ensuring that all voices were heard.

The Walls Come Tumbling Down

Because the members of this interdisciplinary committee, which we call the Performance Improvement Coordinating Group (PICG), knew they were accountable to the Board of Trustees, the medical boards, and administrative leadership about the quality of patient care throughout the entire continuum of care, Quality Management leaders were able to do more than simply identify problems; they could ask why the problems existed and how they should be fixed, and also, they could define a trajectory as to where the organization wanted to go. Quality Management staff moved into the mainstream of integrated patient care, getting out of the regulatory business and into the performance improvement one.

For the first time, various disciplines were regularly brought together in committees to try and interpret and explain the quality data that were made available to them from internal or external sources. Caregivers were encouraged to challenge each other to define best practices and standards of care. Figure 8.3 depicts the lines of communication that enable quality information to flow from the hospital Quality Management Department to the system-level Board of Trustees.

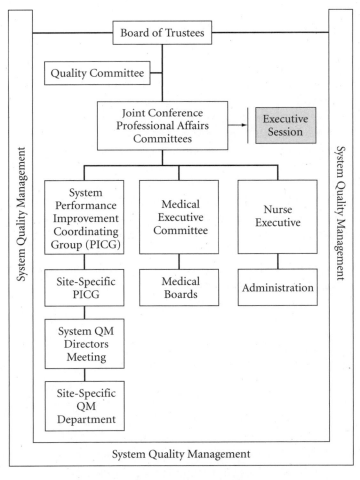

Figure 8.3. Quality Management Lines of Communication.

In this way, the quality assurance model, which identified a problem, asked who did it, and focused only on the responsible party (and always seemed to find one single person to hold responsible), was transformed into a much more sophisticated model where the question was not who made a given error but why it was made, what did the environment contribute to it, and what role leadership played in it. We also asked if this problem was similar to other problems, and if it was possible to fix it, and how. All these variables became key to the analysis. With multiple services involved in the discussion of care, patient safety became the moving force of improvement efforts.

Managing Quality

While Quality Management was developing tools and techniques for performance improvement, the regulatory agencies such as the JCAHO were demanding greater accountability for care from managers and directors, who were expected to define competency and quantify performance in terms of recredentialing criteria and annual employee evaluations. Supervisors were expected to know what was happening on their unit, to identify problems and to understand their nature and frequency, to define their scope of care, to determine if errors were exceptions or typical, and most important, to develop safety nets for improving care and eliminating errors.

Errors were interpreted and analyzed not as isolated events but as part of larger processes. The manager's role was evolving and changing as expectations changed. Managers were becoming more responsible and accountable for identifying common factors on their units in their delivery of care, and for establishing appropriate indicators and developing a methodology to collect and communicate data, to define problems, and to determine solutions to those problems. Managers, in other words, were expected to work within a quality management framework.

Managers were further expected to describe the scope of care on their unit, explain what they did for their patients, outline how they did it, and assess the outcomes of their actions. They were also supposed to know about their patient population (language, ethnicity, age) and the disease processes they handled on their unit, and to aggregate and trend information for use in performance improvement. At departmental meetings, managers reported on the common factors of their patient population, on the common problems facing those patients as shown in data from indicators, and on improvement efforts.

The JCAHO also held health care leadership accountable for performance improvement, and for understanding the rationale, that is, the data and methods behind the improvement efforts. Regulatory standards required that patients be treated with respect and integrity, that there be an articulation of patients' rights and ethics, that treatment be timely and appropriate, and that there be a structure in place to ensure that the organization could provide such standards. The regulatory agencies tried to fill the gap among the administrative and clinical staff, quality methods, and the bedside caregiver. The idea was to eliminate separate and distinct "spheres of influence."

Doing the Right Thing Well

As professionals from various disciplines worked together to establish standards for the delivery of care and to incorporate quality methods into the evaluation of care and performance improvement, it became obvious that compliance with regulatory requirements had to be continuous and not solely for a few days during a survey every three years. Sudden catch-up efforts just wouldn't work. And they shouldn't be necessary—the regulations are designed to protect patient safety constantly.

The administration came to realize the value of maintaining compliance every day and of abiding by the standards and functions of good care. The CEO realized that he was accountable for the provision of care—not just the financial viability of the institution. More important, the CEO understood that when he maintained high standards of quality and mandated the use of quality methodology to evaluate care, the organization benefited financially and the community was more satisfied. Therefore quality management made his job easier.

It was the responsibility of the Quality Management staff to teach others how to speak to the regulatory functions, and that meant learning how to think about care delivery in terms of the regulatory standards and requirements. The Quality Management staff asked managers provocative questions, such as how do you know you are delivering good care or doing a good job or providing good service, since these were the questions asked when the JCAHO surveyed the institution. Managers needed to do more than answer these questions; they had to use data to quantify and prove that they were delivering quality safe care.

They also were expected to understand multidisciplinary performance improvement efforts and the methodology that relied on carefully formulated assumptions, hypotheses, and defined sample size. The JCAHO required that quality improvement, or performance improvement, be accompanied by a narrative that explicitly included a baseline of the care process prior to the performance improvement effort, an explanation of the problem that was being addressed, the composition of the multidisciplinary team that was spearheading the improvement effort, the measurements that were being used to assess and monitor the care, and the outcomes that were being targeted. These expectations helped move the organization toward fully integrating quality into the delivery of care.

Sharing a Common Agenda

Physicians, who were originally reluctant to work within a quality management framework, began to realize the value of relying on quality information and to embrace quality methods when explaining incidents or adverse outcomes that they were required to report to external agencies. Communication between the medical and Quality Management staff improved as the latter mediated between the state and regulatory agencies and the physicians, between the incident or problem and the patient care, and met personally with each physician involved in any case. Physicians realized that Quality Management was the part of the organization that could contribute information about incidents and the physicians' role, and therefore a more integrated relationship between clinicians and Quality Management staff developed. Incident reporting was being handled in a professional and improved manner.

By working together to review an incident, analyzing root causes, outlining flow charts, and developing algorithms regarding adverse outcomes, many disciplines—not just physicians and Quality Management staff—were expected to interact and communicate about the delivery of care that resulted in an incident. And because no one is immune to errors, and thus everyone is vulnerable to having an incident that requires investigation, trust and respect developed between Quality Management and the rest of the organization.

Mutual respect further increased as it became obvious that quality management methodology shared many of the principles of rigorous academic research, in which the medical chairs, in particular, were involved. Medical chairs have a dual role within the hospital; they have administrative responsibilities, juggling resources, and academic responsibilities to do research that involves hypotheses, sample designs, and defined variables—all parallel to the science of quality. As the two disciplines, quality and medicine, discovered that they spoke the same language, communication about the delivery of care improved even further.

Managers were brought into the communication loop because working together—physicians and nurses, managers of various units, and Quality Management—increased the likelihood that care would improve, and patients would have greater satisfaction with the care being delivered. As the traditional silos began to collapse, communication, accountability, and performance improved throughout the organization. Since it is the responsibility of the manager to manage the minute-by-minute care of the doctors' patients, when managers expressed their commitment to providing care with fewer complications to patients, with greater concern for patient safety, and to deliver a positive experience, it became obvious that the managers, the physicians, and the nurses shared a common agenda.

Quality Communication

Managers require superior communication skills to do their job. Nurses and frontline workers are accountable to the needs of their patients, and must answer not only to the physician about the care of individual patients but also to the manager who supervises the care delivered on the unit. Quality management methodology, especially the PDCA, promotes good communication because the expectations of everyone involved, the patient, physician, nurse, and manager, are met. The physician can be confident that care will be provided efficiently and effectively; the nurse will have a framework in which to deliver care in an atmosphere of respect among caregivers and with support from the ancillary staff in an integrated process. The manager will have the objective data necessary to monitor services and enhance improvements. And, most important, the patients will benefit.

For example, how does the manager of a busy and crowded ED oversee the care being delivered? So much is going on all the time. Patients are admitted, many in crisis, by various physicians, all requiring different services; staff turns over every shift. Without processes and procedures in place, chaos reigns and information about the functioning of the unit is lost. However, collecting data, for example, about patients who leave without being evaluated can inform physicians and administration about the flow in the ED. Data regarding readmission to the ED also provide information about the quality of the delivery of care. With objective information, effective policy decisions can be made.

Quality Management Departments have moved out of their metaphorical basement office, where they had minimal staff and even less regard from the medical community; now they are in a position to help shape the organization's destiny as an important component of the strategic planning process. Quality processes and procedures, having proven value, are now integrated into all levels of hospital care, supported by the clear commitment from top administrative and medical leadership. Quality management methods and tools help understand and improve care, and have bridged the isolated silos of nurses, physicians, administrators, and regulatory bodies, forging relationships that result in integrated multidisciplinary teams devoted to performance improvement.

Every supervisor and manager is expected to use quality tools and methods in the monitoring and evaluation of services as well as in improvement efforts. Leadership expects to be informed about data regarding services and the efficient use of resources. Quality information about scope of care and performance improvement is embedded in the job description of managers and supervisors. They are responsible for providing the nursing staff with this education as well. Performance improvement committees and the joint conference committee of the Board of Trustees encompass nurses, chairs of various departments, the quality directors at diverse facilities, clinical and administrative leadership, and together care is evaluated and decisions are made about how to improve care.

The evolution of quality management to incorporate all levels of care, and all disciplines involved in care, took several decades. Change takes time; you'll find no quick way to convince people of your value. But with leadership behind you and with a strong commitment to monitor and assess care, in the aggregate, to understand that care is delivered through processes and not solely by individuals who don't need to communicate with anyone, you will make inroads on the established mindset and patients will be safer in your institution.

SUMMARY

Excellent communication and improved accountability influence the quality of care delivered because of the following factors:

- Health care services are interdependent and involve many departments and services.
- Important information needs to be shared among caregivers.
- Adverse events can be appropriately analyzed for process problems rather than individual failures.
- Data-driven decisions regarding performance improvement require the input of many services.
- Process problems often involve the entire continuum of care.
- Resource efficiency and utilization management need to be integrated into clinical decisions.
- Information regarding appropriate benchmarks for specific disease processes can be aggregated and shared.
- Poor communication can result in adverse events and prolonged and inappropriate utilization of resources.
- Performance improvement involves multidisciplinary teams and analysis of interrelated quality indicators.
- Shared administrative, clinical, and quality goals drive performance.
- Information should be transferred from the bedside to the Board of Trustees.
- Health care providers from various disciplines are accountable to the Board-level multidisciplinary quality committees for providing safe patient care.
- The Board of Trustees expects all health care providers to support quality management methodology for data-driven policy decisions.
- A sophisticated and elaborate committee structure monitors quality care throughout the institution and allows each caregiver a platform to express concerns and priorities.
- Performance improvements require coordination of care among many services and departments.

Things to Think About

- Data show that most stroke patients are ready for discharge home after four or five days, and the clinical literature supports this as well. But physicians are not discharging them until Day 7 or 8.

Describe the different disciplines and staff that would be involved in changing this behavior.

What processes would be targeted for improvement?

When would interventions be necessary in the patient's treatment plan?

• The Board of Trustees at your institution invites you to present a performance improvement plan for your unit or service.

What information do you include in your allotted ten minutes?

How do you report the Board's response back to your staff?

CHAPTER NINE

To Err Is Indeed Human

—⁓— W̶hat would you do if suddenly your unit was plunged into darkness, and the entire hospital was without electrical power? No air conditioning, no lights, no ventilators, no technological or critical monitoring devices, no way for people trapped in elevators to get out, no water, no refrigeration, no computers or electrically dependent services of any kind. A massive power failure—an incident over which you have no control—could be disastrous. How would your unit manage? Would your patients be safe and well cared for?

How would you react to such an event? You could follow the steps required for safe patient evacuation or you could look for the emergency generator or you could do nothing at all and hope that someone else would manage the problem before anything too awful happened. Such incidents can and do occur, and managers have to be prepared to deal with them. We would like to use our collective experience over the years managing crises to outline some of the factors involved in coping with serious events. We will use hypothetical events since actual events are protected by New York State law.

MANAGING CRISES

The impact of an incident such as a power failure can be tremendous, affecting every service in the institution, disrupting the delivery of care, and reminding the managers of all departments how important it is to protect their patients, understand their environment, have contingency plans and processes in place in case of emergency, test equipment effectively, and train staff to think critically and react appropriately in a crisis. The midst of a crisis is no time to invent a backup process or to institute policies to protect patients. The nature of an emergency is that routine care stops until the crisis is managed, unless you have had the forethought to put plans and practice into place—for use in the event of an emergency.

An environmental incident such as a power failure serves to focus attention on the importance of understanding every detail of the care delivered on every unit. If you press a button and nothing happens, what do you do? Whose responsibility is it to ensure that everything works properly? What is the maintenance schedule for equipment checks? What emergency plans are available? As a manager, you may be removed from the technical aspects of the problem, but you are still accountable to your patients and responsible for ensuring that the technical staff provide proper support to your unit. Part of your job is to oversee the environment.

Understanding What Happened

Assume that the power really did go out. Analysis of such an incident can take a great deal of time and involve many people. Remember that the point of doing an analysis of an incident is not only to understand and alleviate a problem but also to ensure that in the future such a situation would be better managed or eliminated altogether. What if the investigation revealed that the local power company had been doing emergency repairs on the power line that fed the hospital and took it out of operation without alerting the hospital in advance? Even worse, when the power was disrupted, the hospital's emergency generators failed to engage. Such an incident can provide a serious wake-up call to a hospital, which is the reason the JCAHO requires an evaluation and a maintenance program for emergency power. Was this hospital in compliance with that regulation?

Using Quality Analysis Tools

To investigate the causes of this event, a multidisciplinary team, including an engineering consultant, reviewed the factors involved. As illustrated in Figure 9.1, a cause-and-effect analysis identified a host of factors all contributing to a poor outcome.

For example, the generator was inaccessible and the backup generators had not been tested under conditions that adequately simulated a real power outage. Emergency equipment that was necessary to keep patients safe was not readily available for staff to use. Furthermore, the leadership response was poor; no one seemed to know what to do. Managers from various departments had not been appropriately trained in disaster planning. Staffing was insufficient to handle the crisis and there was a delay in securing the building. Other staff involved in this incident were inadequately educated about how to react to protect patients in the event of this type of emergency. Several members of the engineering staff did not work directly for the hospital; they were contract employees who were unfamiliar with hospital processes and procedures, and they had no policies for servicing the equipment.

External factors also had an impact on the problem. Communication from the power authority to the health system was poor. Although multiple community agencies responded to the event, it was unclear who should be in charge. Vendors with the job of ensuring that the equipment was properly maintained were not competently managed and their work was slipshod.

In performing a root cause analysis (RCA), the investigative team wrestled with a series of increasingly specific questions that drill down through the causes of an event to uncover the fundamental flaws in the process. What happened? Why did it happen? What were the factors that could have been controlled? What factors were beyond control? What services were implicated? What processes underlay the failure of equipment and personnel? Was staffing adequate in number and competency to handle the situation that resulted? What information should have been communicated? Were leadership responsibilities effectively carried out? Who was responsible? How could the problems be corrected?

As the team collected responses regarding the questions asked, more questions surfaced. Managers are expected not to be satisfied until all the whys have been answered; and if the answer is unknown,

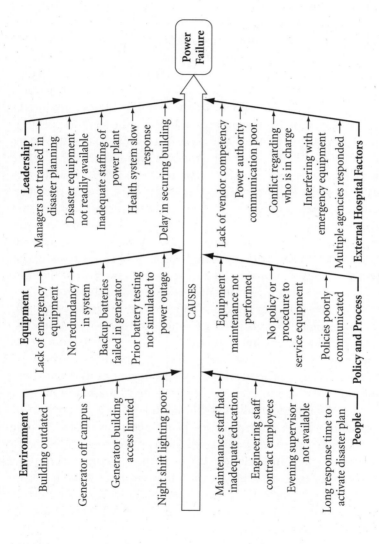

Figure 9.1. Cause-and-Effect Analysis: Power Outage.

that is also important. Why does no one have the answer? Who should? What information would be required to answer the question?

The RCA of the power outage described here would drill down through the factors identified in the cause-and-effect analysis. For example, the failure in preventive maintenance relating to the testing of the batteries in the backup generators meant that the batteries were not charged up when the outage occurred. No one had any process, procedure, or accountability for monitoring the condition of the batteries. Hospital staff believed the equipment was being properly maintained, and therefore they did not anticipate the potential for disaster.

This incident underlines how necessary it is for the manager's role to extend beyond the unit and even the hospital, reaching out into the community so that connections between the community and the institution can be maintained. Since incidents can involve community resources, fostering such relationships is very beneficial: police are involved in traffic control; the fire department supplies emergency generators. As manager, you need to know who to contact, and if you have established a relationship when things are calm, in a crisis you will be able to reach out to the appropriate person and not start introducing yourself while an emergency erupts around you. Such relationships are valuable in routine care and in crises as well. If, as an example, you manage an ED, then trauma patients are brought to you via fire department and local ambulance service. Having a relationship with these groups may provide for a smoother admission for these patients.

Returning to the example, the analysis also revealed a lack of accountability in this event. It was unclear who was supposed to be responsible for monitoring the batteries in the generator. Unless this responsibility is clearly defined elsewhere, it is the manager's responsibility. The manager should have communicated to the Engineering Department through the Hospital Safety Committee or the Performance Improvement Committees to ensure a safe environment for the patients.

Proactive Analysis

In addition to doing a root cause analysis of a particular event that has occurred, a failure mode and effects analysis (FMEA) should be conducted. This time-consuming analysis attempts to identify which points in a process might be vulnerable to failure. Once the risks are identified, the multidisciplinary team tries to evaluate how often each process might fail, what would be the severity of the effect of the failure, and whether any detection routines are in place to alert caregivers that the process has failed.

The major difference between these two kinds of analyses is that the RCA is reactive and used to analyze an unwanted outcome, whereas the FMEA is proactive and takes a prospective look at processes to try and identify risk points and problems with the goal of establishing preventive measures so that patient safety is maintained (see Figure 9.2).

With both the RCA and the FMEA, the end result is an action plan that provides recommendations about improving processes. As the Joint Commission Perspectives on Patient Safety (March 2003) points out, in an RCA one asks *why* something happened; with an FMEA, one asks *what if* this happened, how would we respond, and how could we respond better? Since errors are by and large caused by good people who are well intentioned and well trained, RCA and FMEA focus on processes, usually assessing the impact of technology, staffing, and leadership. Another way to think about the difference between the

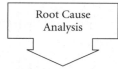

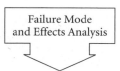

- Reacts to events

- Retrospective review

- Asks, "What happened?"

- Determine what factors have an impact on the problem

- Adverse outcome is defined

- Helps determine risk points and corrective actions

- Corrective action plan provides recommendation about improving process

- Anticipates risk points

- Prospective analysis

- Asks, "What if this happened?"

- Anticipates outcome

- Examine process to identify vulnerabilities and flaws

- Preventive strategies proved recommendation about improving process

**Figure 9.2.   Comparison Between Root Cause
Analysis and Failure Mode and Effects Analysis.**

two analyses is that in an RCA, you examine the adverse incident to determine what factors had an impact on it, and in an FMEA, you examine an entire process rather than an outcome of that process in an effort to identify vulnerabilities and flaws.

When you do an RCA or FMEA, select a team to perform the analysis from as many services, departments, and disciplines as you think relevant to garner as much information as possible and recognize various concerns and points of view. Once an initial analysis is complete, it is the team's responsibility to communicate results to the rest of the institution. Sharing information serves to educate others about the faulty process and about the improvements being proposed.

Analysis of an event such as a power outage that has an impact on patient care is the most intelligent response a manager can make. Mistakes will happen; they always do. Our experience has made it clear that the best course of action is to face a mistake head on. Often, the first impulse is to duck a problem, especially if you think it will not directly affect patient care. But sooner or later all problems have an impact. Attention to the process, in the form of an FMEA, can reveal failures in the delivery of care that are not readily apparent during the daily routine of work.

Process Improvements

The purpose of either the RCA or the FMEA is to introduce improvements, not only for a single unit but across the entire continuum of care. In this example, the policy for competency needed to be redefined because it was necessary to clarify what was expected from outside vendors who provide maintenance services to the institution. The manager's job includes supervising vendor competency and education regarding policies and procedures because the manager is responsible for setting expectations for outside agents who provide services and affect care on the unit. Another weakness that the analysis revealed was that in the event of a power failure, ventilator-dependent patients required special maintenance. An improvement that could be initiated would be to have EMS available for transport and to help with ventilator patients and suction.

What is especially interesting about this kind of global event is that all the managers in every department are challenged to be responsible for the environmental factors on their own units. They are forced to analyze their care in terms of safety for patients, to identify what in the environment could cause harm, and to develop contingency plans that not only address the technologies affected by an event like a power outage but also assign and educate staff for accountability.

For example, timing can be crucial if the event disrupts some kind of critical process or service such as a ventilator. Whose job is it to come running? Or if defibrillators can't work, what is the backup plan? Managers need to understand the equipment involved in their patients' care and to have a real command of alternatives.

As a manager, you manage more than people and processes; you also manage equipment and the environment of care. It may sound trivial, but it is extremely important to know where the flashlights are and to keep the batteries alive and to know if the emergency phones work. In other words, to maintain safety of the patient in the bed, even for those patients who are not on power-dependent equipment, the entire environment should be proactively protected. Until you deliberately analyze your processes, either through an RCA or an FMEA, the elements of a corrective action or performance improvement initiative are obscure.

LEARNING FROM MISTAKES

Bedside care that has evolved around evidence-based medicine, guidelines, clinical pathways, and policies and procedures is not designed to dictate what is derogatorily referred to as "cookbook medicine." On the contrary, these processes have been established to avoid mistakes. The diversity of care that has to be managed, the variation in technology, the complexity of medication, and the varied patient population, all require order and routine. A caregiver might skip a step in the process of care or take a shortcut that does not cause harm to one patient, but the next patient might be different, or skipping another step might have a negative impact on care. One of the great values of an FMEA is that it increases awareness about process problems and shortcuts that have a potential impact on care.

Events and errors provide opportunities to learn about the flaws in underlying processes, so that future similar events can be avoided. That is the premise of both the RCA and the FMEA. When supervisors and managers analyze problems rather than simply blame the person nearest to the incident, they generally find process problems that need to be addressed, human factors issues that focus attention on staffing numbers and competency, environmental concerns that were not considered, and the like.

Almost without exception, however, the study of errors through RCA or FMEA reveals failures of communication, which is one of the most critical issues a manager or supervisor has to cope with. You want to do everything in your power to eliminate risks and avoid errors—for the patient and for the institution. Incidents can cause terrible damage to patients, and if an adverse event is publicized, programs and reputations that were created over time can be destroyed in a single day.

Communication Problems

It is a wise manager who is able to consider individual caregivers as members of a larger caregiving team, a group working within a flawed process. For individuals to function as an effective team, however, communication among members must be encouraged. For example, in an operating room many specialists from various disciplines must work in an integrated and complementary manner for the patient to be properly managed. These specialists know what is expected of them, and they know what to expect from one another. They are trained to recognize a crisis and respond accordingly to minimize harm to the patient and complete the procedure.

When surgical errors occur, analysis reveals again and again that poor communication was a primary cause. Sometimes the surgeon is aloof and refuses to act as part of a team. With that link broken, communication fails and the team fractures, and the patient is put at risk. In addition, if the group does not function as a unified team, when a member suspects or realizes that an error is occurring, fear or intimidation can cause that person to fail to communicate. Terrible consequences can result, including unexpected death.

It falls to the manager to educate the surgeons to function as part of a team and to encourage open communication from the rest of the team as well. For a nurse to remind a surgeon that the CAT scan should be used to verify the operative site prior to the first incision could be very intimidating in the traditional hospital culture that defines the two roles as separate and unequal. The manager's job is to create an environment in the OR (or any other unit) that can reduce intimidation. If individuals on a team have a single goal in mind, that is, to promote the patient's well-being and not their own specific agendas, intimidation will not be an issue.

Technology Problems

Giving blood to a patient via transfusion is a common procedure but one that carries a high risk for the patient who receives the wrong blood. Proper patient identification is crucial to the delivery of compatible blood, and health care workers therefore have elaborate processes and procedures, supported by computer technology, to ensure that the correct blood is delivered to the correct patient.

Managers should be aware of the issues involved in providing the right patient with the correct blood in the appropriate volume. Being alert to potential problems allows the manager to take steps to avoid incidents and preserve patient safety. As blood travels from the blood bank to the patient, many disciplines and personnel are involved, increasing the risk for errors. Because of the high volume and high risk of this procedure, unit managers, the managers of the blood bank, the nursing staff, and the Quality Management Department should form a team to examine the processes involved on an ongoing basis to eliminate potential problems. Stagnant processes are vulnerable processes.

Imagine an incident where an unforeseen problem such as a lethal computer virus causes the servers to crash, leaving the entire hospital without computer technology. Although it has auxiliary processes to handle manually what is usually done technically, it has neither tested nor used these processes in many years. Will they go smoothly? Probably not. In such high-risk environments as the blood bank, drills should be conducted regularly to determine that the processes are effective.

The consequences of the computer crash might include the following scenario. In the blood bank, the technician pulled the wrong blood bag, partly because he was so used to the computer verifying that the blood matched the order that he failed to confirm that the blood type was that of the patient. He was out of practice when it came to relying on his own intelligence, so his vigilance was lax. He handed the blood bag to the transporter, who signed for it automatically, acknowledging only that she had picked up the order rather than doing the cross-check she was expected to do regarding the accuracy of every batch of blood (type, match, identification) she was transporting. Since mistakes were never made in the computerized system, she was also negligent.

The nurse who administered the blood and the second nurse who was supposed to confirm the accuracy of the blood match (as per the required procedure) were also behaving in a rote manner, assuming that since the blood bank always sent up the correct blood and since no red flags had been raised when the blood left the blood bank, it would be correct in this instance also. The confirming nurse trusted the administering nurse because he knew her to be very competent; therefore, if she was hanging the blood, it was the right blood to be hanging. In other words, none of the people involved in the complex blood transfusion process, from the blood bank, transport, and nursing, followed the detailed procedures that had been developed to check for accuracy in terms of blood-patient identification. Nor did they communicate effectively with each other—because ever since the computers took on the job, they'd had little need for careful and precise interpersonal communication.

In an interesting way, relying on technology, which is supposed to override human error, can cause humans to err. Machines fail. People have to be prepared to do their jobs with extra care in the face of technological problems, which means that they always have to be well prepared. Technology makes our lives easier, especially in the busy and complex environment of delivery of care at the bedside, but technology provides only support; caregivers provide care.

Relying on technology can have serious consequences. The delivery of the wrong blood as described here could be missed entirely if the patient had no adverse reaction. The error might have been discovered only when the computers were repaired and reacted to the discrepancy between the order and the blood taken from the blood bank. Remember that if the patient has an adverse reaction to the administration of incorrect blood, as is common, the physician who ordered the blood, the team involved in the process, and the managers from all the relevant services are held accountable, never the computer. Technology is designed to assist people at their jobs, not replace them.

Managers have to be confident that their staff will respond appropriately to maintain patient safety in the event of a technological failure. Our reliance on computers can blind us to their limitations. For example, at a system in another part of the country, when the computers failed, the Pharmacy programs were damaged so that when the computers came back up, the computers started spewing incorrect medication orders. Hundreds of people received incorrect prescriptions before someone noticed the error. Despite the movement to incorporate more and more technology into health care delivery, computers are no substitute for human intelligence and critical thinking by well-trained and competent people.

Implementing Change

You don't need to wait for an error to occur to implement change on your unit. You can learn from the errors of other institutions and set up protective policies and procedures or relevant education for your staff. The JCAHO and other organizations dedicated to patient safety, such as the Agency for Healthcare Research and Quality and the National Patient Safety Foundation, share information about errors so that institutions can take precautions to avoid similar ones. The media also report on errors so that the public can have the advantage of information.

Recently, at a sophisticated and renowned teaching hospital, a young patient receiving a liver transplant died because of being given incompatible blood. In another recent case, at another prestigious institution, the laboratory mixed up the identification of the mother's and father's blood, identifying the father as the suitable donor when in fact it was the mother. Their child died. No end of similar errors could be cited, but the point of these two is that both were avoidable and would not have occurred had there been vigilant protective processes in place. As a manager, you don't want to wait for a crisis to analyze your processes.

Any medical process that involves many people—and what medical process today doesn't?—carries with it the potential for error. If we haven't said it enough times already, safety and competency depend on clear areas of accountability and improved and clear communication. If you value and encourage critical thinking in your staff, your staff will step up to the plate in an emergency, which is precisely what you hope for.

Anticipate Problems

The recognition of risk points in the complex process of blood delivery caused us to examine it in detail. A multidisciplinary group of physicians, nurses, staff from the blood bank, from Transport, and relevant managers from across the hospital met over a period of months. Smaller groups discussed the process used at different environments in the hospital, trying to identify risk points and best practices. For each environment, explicit and exact procedures were in place for the ordering, identification, transport, and delivery of blood. It was crucial to identify what could prevent these processes from being followed. The conclusions from the analysis are relevant to many processes in addition to blood delivery.

It is human nature to try and circumvent obstacles and also to find the line of least resistance in any activity. The analysis revealed that informal processes were beginning to replace the more formal ones, and that there was a fine line between routinizing a process so that in case of emergency everyone reacts automatically to do the right thing and making a process so routine that people stop thinking or find creative ways to circumvent the process or adapt it to their own requirements, thereby changing and personalizing it. In high-risk processes and procedures, routines may be very helpful, but less risky cases should have some room for individual creativity so that individuals need to think to work effectively and safely. The manager of the unit must constantly observe the employees' performance as well as patients' reaction to treatment to identify any issues that might result in negative outcomes.

If you can identify the gap between formal and informal behavior in a complex process, you can make progress toward making that gap smaller. You can't expect human beings not to act like human beings. For example, imagine a scenario where Transport picked up blood at lunchtime. The person is responsible and has been trained that blood should not be brought into an area other than the ones it is supposed to, certainly not into the cafeteria. But people get hungry and want to eat. What do they do with the blood while they are eating? This is the kind of problem that an FMEA can expose for analysis.

Or another example: a very competent and experienced nurse put a vial of blood in her pocket, meaning to label it with the correct name when the computer-generated label came up to the unit. But it never happened. For some reason processing the label was delayed. The nurse had drawn the blood but had no label to affix. What to do? Such simple questions, if analyzed in advance, can avoid an incident. Relying on memory is never a good idea. But the discrepancy in timing between drawing the blood and receiving the printout of the label has to be addressed somehow. What were the options available for the nurse? In a better process, what could be developed? Perhaps something as easy as having labels available for writing with pen—just in case—would do the job.

An FMEA can productively bring many such process flaws to a manager's attention. For example, how could processes be improved to address the situation of two individuals in the ED with similar or even the same name? Bloods are drawn on both and one's lab results reveal the need for a transfusion. Is there a process in place to avoid confusion?

Another example of a process problem that can be highlighted during a proactive FMEA: During a particularly bloody surgery, a physician uses a towel to absorb the blood and inadvertently leaves the towel in the patient's abdomen. Using the towel was a deviation from the normal procedure but there was no process to manage this deviation, although it is widely recognized that these types of ad hoc actions can occur. Even a count policy wouldn't have helped here because towels are not counted, only pads.

Doing an FMEA might lead to a policy that eliminates towels from the OR, or makes sure that towels are routinely counted, or, perhaps most simply, that the surgeon announces the deviation from normal practice to the other staff in the room to establish shared responsibility for remembering that something out of the ordinary has occurred and has to be managed at the end of the procedure to ensure that all equipment is accounted for. There is no single right answer. But the attempt to analyze a process and anticipate possible risks to patient safety and implement strategies to avoid them can prevent tragedy.

MANAGING ERRORS

Errors will always occur. You need to expect them, prepare for them, and have a process in place to deal with them, so you are not reacting to each event as a unique crisis. Take nothing for granted. You want your staff committed to minimizing the possibility of mistakes and to competently identifying risk points and taking sensible precautions against them. You and your staff need to actively communicate about errors and the potential for errors. Part of your job is to manage errors—that means to supervise people, processes, and the environment, to analyze and become informed about the reasons for the error, to implement improvements to avoid future errors, to define and monitor appropriate documentation addressing the error, to supervise the medical care of the patient, to interact with the other professionals involved in the error and with the patient's family, and to consider the ethical issues and possibly even legal problems that might arise from the error. All this requires communication.

Talking About Errors

It is vitally important for you to encourage an open and free flow of communication, not only among your staff but also between staff members and the patient and family. Research reveals that when patients and caregivers communicate in an open and honest way, and when facts are not obscured but explained by people willing to cooperate to understand any deviation from the standard of care, patients are much less likely to litigate or to complain, even in the face of serious errors.

Patients want to be told the truth, regardless of whether or not the truth reveals that poor judgment was used or that inadequate care was delivered. Telling it straight really is doing the right thing. But to do that, you have to admit that a problem occurred, and you have to admit it not only to yourself and to your staff but also to the patient and family—and you have to acquire information about what actually occurred. Patients often deserve apologies, and rarely is a caregiver comfortable offering one. Often, when an error has occurred in the delivery of care, the patient suspects it. Telling the truth is not only respectful and ethical, it also allows the patient to participate as a partner in the process of care, which generally results in improved outcomes.

Since errors cannot be totally eliminated and since staff are usually not eager to run to you with information about their mistakes, part of your job as a manager is to find a way to best identify and to analyze those errors that do occur, with the goal of learning from them and making improvements. Everything we have discussed thus far—the importance of communication and accountability, using clinical guidelines, understanding performance in a detailed way, using the PDCA to make improvements, and basing your evaluation of care on measurements—is involved in managing and analyzing errors.

Know Your Environment

In health care—it cannot be said too often—errors will inevitably occur; there are just too many variables to control. Medical care is delivered by human beings to human beings, people who may be stressed and pressured and rushed and tired and distracted or even incompetent, who may have language issues or social issues that make an impact on care delivery and inhibit communication. Patients also may have all kinds of complicating factors, comorbidities, education levels, and demographic and cultural profiles that interfere with perfect care, or unique physiological and psychological characteristics that influence treatment and outcomes. Therefore, being aware of risks and alert to the potential for mistakes is good management.

Some administrative and medical leaders talk about achieving "zero defect," that is, creating an environment where mistakes will never happen, and where every step along the delivery of care is perfect. It would certainly be nice if you could insist on and expect perfect practices and procedures from your staff and thus eliminate any errors in judgment or mistakes. But zero defect, although a worthy goal, is unrealistic in a health care setting. What may work in a factory, or in the manufacture of objects, doesn't readily translate to the complexity of people caring for people. Think about a car assembly line of the type introduced by Henry Ford. Everyone has a small piece of the larger project they can perfect. They do the same thing the same way day after day. The tools and the processes of manufacturing inanimate objects allow for a great deal of uniformity and standardization, and that permits uniform expectations of excellence.

On the classic assembly line, communication is minimal. Crucial information does not have to be processed or shared. A dozen people are not all focused on a single procedure, sometimes under tremendous pressure. The goal of car production, for example, is for each car to be identical to all the other cars of that model coming off the line. Cars can be produced with zero defects. However, a patient, when discharged, is entirely unique and individual. Although every effort should be made to make the hospital environment as risk-free and as safe as possible, and health care institutions and the individuals who work in them need to work to eliminate errors to the degree possible, a hospital is simply not a factory and should never be considered one.

Safety First

Finding ways to eliminate medical errors is very much in the news these days, having come to the forefront of public attention following media exposure of errors that have occurred, and of medical groups such as the IOM that have reported that medical errors kill more than ninety-eight thousand patients yearly. Government agencies are holding health care institutions explicitly accountable for patient safety, which is a relatively recent phenomenon. The public recognition of errors puts hospitals and caregivers on notice. Patients expect a safe environment and excellent results.

What goes a long way toward improving safety and reducing risk is the consciousness that deviation from developed protocols may harm patients in unanticipated ways. Using the quality process to examine and monitor effectiveness of care, the manager can target patient safety in the most ordinary care processes. Regulatory agencies require hospitals to focus on adverse events and on creating methodologies to prevent their occurrence. For example, medication, one of the most common treatments administered in a hospital, is a frequent source of harm to patients.

Recommendations from private groups to medical societies advocate a paperless, computerized process to eliminate many of these errors. The rationale is that computers would override deviation from the standard of care that occurs due to human error. However, even with computer use, errors still occur. Managers must understand the medication process from prescription to administration, develop processes to minimize risk to patients, and collect data on an ongoing basis regarding medication delivery.

Effective 2004, the JCAHO has identified seven patient safety goals that health care institutions have to improve: accuracy of patient identification; effectiveness of communication among caregivers; safety of using high-alert medications; elimination of wrong site, wrong patient, wrong procedure surgery; improvements to the safety of infusion pumps and the effectiveness of clinical alarms; and reduce the risk of health care–acquired infections. The scope and range of these safety goals indicate the scope and range of the errors reported.

These patient safety goals impose consciousness regarding risk factors on these very common processes. The reason the Joint Commission has made improving processes for verbal orders, for example, a national safety goal is that numerous patients were harmed through problems associated with verbal orders. When physicians use the telephone or say orders rather than write them in the chart, everyone involved has to be conscious of the resulting risks to the patient. If the transcribers don't hear well, or they misunderstand the order, they may specify the incorrect medication or dosage. Managers are encouraged to use such reports to think about these problems and develop policies and safety measures. Should high-risk medications never be ordered over the telephone? If so, who is accountable for monitoring that the physicians abide by the new policy?

Defining Error

The definition of what constitutes a medical error is so culture-bound that it changes as attitudes change. Before this push for patient safety and institutional accountability, errors were defined solely by physicians. What were considered tolerable errors were more egregious mistakes than what we would accept today. Until this recent focus on patient safety, errors were regarded as a normal and expected, if unfortunate, part of the delivery of care. The attitude was that sometimes things didn't work out the way they should, which was of course lamentable, but . . .

In other words, mistakes were not really considered, labeled, defined, or understood as errors, as events to analyze and prevent. Errors were not thought to be institutional or the result of poor procedures but rather were considered to be physician-specific. Quality leader Dr. Ernest Codman was prescient regarding errors. As long ago as 1890 he had the perspective, mostly unshared by the medical profession, that poor outcomes were the result of errors or mistakes and should not be excused as the result of tolerable subjective judgment.

Mistakes were discussed as part of the routine physician peer review process (M&M), and characterized as normal complications. The occasional poor outcome was accepted, especially if the patient was in the care of an inexperienced physician who would learn over time. If an experienced physician made a mistake (which of course also occurred), well, it had to be understood in context. That physician had done thousands and thousands of procedures and only had one or two errors among them. Luckily for all of us, the times they are a-changing.

Today, the definition of an error that must be addressed is very broad. It isn't necessary for the patient to have a bad outcome for some process or treatment to be considered an error. An error focuses on the care delivered, regardless of its impact on the patient. For example, if a patient received a medication that shouldn't have been given, that is an error in the delivery of care, whether or not the patient had a reaction.

Analyzing Potential Errors

With this broader definition of error, managers can use analysis of near misses to great advantage to improve processes without patient endangerment. When one of our tertiary hospitals instituted a blame-free reporting form for medication errors—a form that did not re-quire identification of the person involved—reports of near misses in-creased. Nurses were encouraged to report all minor incidents so that processes and environments could be evaluated for safety.

Those reports were analyzed and as a result, for example, certain medications were taken off the units and other safeguards were im-plemented at the Pharmacy. Happily the awareness of the safety risk did not involve an incident to a patient. Perhaps, through the aware-ness of the vulnerability in the system, some lives were saved. At a community hospital, Pharmacy Department staff began monitoring and measuring their interventions, those instances where they caught a potential error. They found almost seven hundred near misses a month! Aggregating the data and analyzing those areas most vulner-able to errors helped the hospital improve processes. As a manager, you'll find striving for increased reporting of near misses worthwhile, as it could eliminate unwanted and unexpected errors.

For example, perhaps on your unit, which is understaffed, a nurse delivers aspirin to a patient later than was scheduled. The nurse might have been prioritizing apparently more critical medications and de-livering the aspirin only after all the others. Is this a serious problem? Would you define not giving aspirin on time as a near miss, a poten-tially harmful event? It is up to the manager to define an error in the delivery of service on that particular unit, including potential errors, and to communicate that definition and concept to the staff. In this case an error of omission (rather than commission), not giving meds in a timely way, might be considered an error.

Small problems grow into big ones. Delayed delivery of aspirin is a small problem that might alert the manager to potentially bigger problems: being understaffed, or having too many medications deliv-ered at the same time, or facing some other bottleneck in the process that should be fixed. It is possible that aspirin not taken on time could have side effects, including pain, that could lead to other problems. If the goal is to eliminate potential crises before they occur, the best way to do that is to deal with small problems before they become big ones.

Think of those people who build airplanes. The worker who turns a certain screw a certain way may one day take a shortcut, for what-ever reason, and not turn it fully or make it tight enough. This seems like an entirely trivial occurrence, but incident analysis has made us aware that it is precisely something as seemingly insignificant as a loose screw that could cause a plane to crash, killing many people. It pays to deal with little problems as if they could have big effects.

If a plane crash was analyzed through an RCA, and the fact that the technician took a shortcut when tightening the screw was uncovered, the manufacturer might make certain corrective actions regarding reeducation or process reviews as a result of this event. However, if the manager conducted an FMEA about the process of assembling planes, and examined how often certain shortcuts were taken and why and how it might be possible to avoid those shortcuts in future, a more extensive corrective action could be considered. It pays to see the drawbacks in a process before one of them results in an incident.

Therefore, it is good management to develop processes to review and analyze issues on your unit before big problems arise. Do an FMEA. Bring the staff together for a staff meeting to discuss the issues surrounding medication delivery, including aspirin. Ask them for suggestions about how to improve. Perhaps it is an HR staffing issue, and you have to deal with floaters, nurses who are untrained for the specific job they are doing, or day workers who haven't had the appropriate orientation to their responsibilities, or there is such a shortage of staff that nurses are pulled from one unit to another. Or it could be a Pharmacy issue, where the medications are not delivered in a timely way, or there is not enough control of high-risk medications. Or the nurse is overloaded working overtime as a result of staffing problems. Use the PDCA. The role of quality management, and what it has to offer, is the use of information to teach, define, educate, and measure performance for improvement.

It's Never One Thing

Errors that occur during the medication delivery process are unfortunately quite common, being among the top sentinel events reported throughout the country. A medication error often reveals multiple opportunities for improvement—something that is easily understandable if one considers how many people, at various levels of competency, and how many processes, from the writing of the prescription to the actual administration, are involved in the typical medication process illustrated in Figure 9.3.

Risk points are obvious at all the critical steps, including the prescribing, preparation, dispensing, and administration phases. Physicians outside the hospital grounds can use the telephone to call in medication orders, which are frequently misunderstood, which is why the JCAHO has included verbal orders in its recent safety goals. In most errors, communication is found to be a major factor.

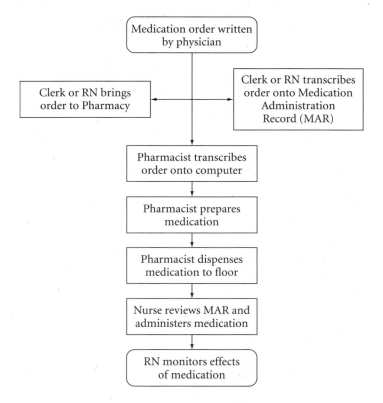

Figure 9.3.   Flow Chart: Medication Delivery Process.

Root cause analyses can usually identify multiple human factors issues implicated in a medication error. Personality characteristics— shyness, individual perceptions and expectations, moods, arrogance— all have an impact on communication and can shape interactions and lead to an event. Even when everyone means well, the process is so complex that it is vulnerable to error.

Imagine a case where a resident ordered a drug based on assessment and after consultation with an attending physician. Being unfamiliar with the drug, the resident checked two sources for verification of dosage and wrote the order, but misspelled the drug and wrote the time of administration unclearly. The nurse who received the order was also unfamiliar with the drug and transcribed the handwritten version with the wrong time of administration and the wrong spelling of the drug.

A second nurse, to whom the first turned for advice, did not know the drug and attempted to use the reference guide, without results, but did not ask anyone else for help. After performing an incorrect mathematical calculation regarding the appropriate dosage for the patient, the second nurse called the Pharmacy to order the drug. The pharmacist misread the nurse's uncertainty as urgency and sent the requested medication to the unit in an undiluted, concentrated form. At the bedside, the first nurse prepared the syringe, disregarding two warning labels that indicated that the drug must be diluted, and labeled the syringe incorrectly, according to what had been ordered rather than what had actually arrived.

In addition, as is often the case, the event occurred during a vulnerable time period—when the shift changed for both nursing and resident staff. An increased workload in the ICU necessitated additional coverage from the original resident, who was also covering another unit. This young doctor was unable to complete the administration of the medication, as the process from ordering to administration took over an hour, and she was required to finish her coverage on the other unit. Therefore, a second resident was called in to administer the medication, and asked the second nurse about the dose. The nurse replied with the incorrect number, and the resident administered the drug without checking the accuracy of the high-risk order. Rather than delivering the drug as an IV drip, the resident mistakenly administered the entire dose in one concentrated infusion. The overdose resulted in cardiac arrest to the patient.

Miscommunication occurred throughout this situation. The pharmacist believed that the drug was required urgently and so sent it to the unit in undiluted form, assuming that the nurse was familiar with the use of the drug and would dilute it properly before administration. The nurse didn't feel comfortable questioning the physician or pharmacist about how to calculate the correct dose for the drip, and failed to use available resources such as the charge nurse or nurse educator. The nurse also did not make use of the reference guide for medication, which would have been informative about the correct use of this drug. The resident did not question the attending physician about a drug with which she was unfamiliar.

In addition to their lack of communication (as well as their miscommunication), the participants displayed a lack of competency and critical thinking skills, especially with regard to the calculation of the appropriate dosage, and of the form of administration, whether to deliver the medication via a slow drip or by quick infusion. They also failed to adhere to policy and procedures of medication administration. High-risk drugs are not supposed to be dispensed from the Pharmacy in undiluted form.

This medication error was the result of multiple failures, with a confluence of circumstances that began a set of dominoes' toppling. No one was watching carefully enough or was accountable for stopping the collapse. That's an indication of poor management. The social environment, its organizational structure, mode of communication, and perception about mutual roles at the bedside contributed significantly to the error. This incident involved more than a nurse or physician. Entire processes should be reviewed and revamped for all critical care areas in the hospital and wherever medication delivery is emergent.

MANAGING INCIDENTS

Occurrences that do not result in serious injury are reported internally; incidents that involve harm to patients are required to be reported to state and regulatory agencies, which means that the manager has to be well informed about the causes of the incident and prepared to develop corrective actions. Many managers do not realize that the investigation required to complete the paperwork involved in incident reporting is a wonderful opportunity to explore processes and develop improvements. Often individuals are intimidated by the depth of detail required, or trained to offer only minimal facts about a case to the outside world. We would encourage everyone involved in an incident to report it in the most analytical detail possible.

Reporting Incidents

Regardless of the severity of the incident, analysis should be performed—even with an event that did not cause patient harm, processes may be so flawed that the next time a similar incident could have a more severe outcome. As manager, you don't want to have any incidents, even if they were not serious. Therefore you need to proactively analyze and implement improvements. If, for example, a visitor reports that a patient has fallen, you need to investigate. Were there witnesses? Was the patient alone? What is the patient's history? What factors contributed? Part of the unit manager's responsibility is to train staff to adequately and informatively fill in an occurrence report.

When a serious event does occur, the manager should immediately take action. First inform your manager to say that you will be absorbed in an inquiry, then contact the Quality Management Department, who will help you with the mandatory reports for the external agencies. To complete these reports, you need a great deal of information. Investigation should begin at once. Incidents need to be analyzed quickly so that memory is fresh, records are located, and corrections to a faulty process or education regarding a good process can be accelerated to avoid repetition of the incident.

Our state defines which errors are serious enough to be reported (for example, a surgical error that resulted in patient harm, a fall that results in fracture, a surgical wound infection) and those that require root cause analysis (such as wrong site surgery, retained foreign body, unexpected death due to inappropriate care). Generally, RCA must be done on any unexpected adverse occurrence that was not directly related to the patient's illness or underlying condition. The framework that the state uses and that of the JCAHO is quite similar, both for what constitutes a serious event and what kinds of questions to ask to discover how that event happened.

The level of detail required means that the manager has to be very well informed about the incident. If you were not directly involved in the incident, this requires serious detective work. Interview everyone. Ask why and listen carefully to the answers. Assess the patient's condition following the event. Consider if staffing was adequate and if the environment contributed. Was a policy in place, or does one need to be developed? Is the staff informed about the policy? If there was a policy, and the staff knew it, was it followed? If not, why not? What kinds of shortcuts were taken? All this is the responsibility of the manager: to educate staff regarding policies and procedures, to ensure adequate staffing, to monitor the environment of care. Was the unit effectively managed, with sophisticated organization and strict expectations as to appropriate roles? A lax environment breeds errors because it leaves so much care to chance.

Talk to experts, including physicians, about the procedures involved in the occurrence. Ask what should have happened that didn't. The manager is expected to put all the facts together and determine how processes, medications, equipment, communication, and so on, interacted to cause the event. Never assume anything—including that the most logical explanation is the correct one. Keep an open mind and look at all the factors surrounding the case.

When doing a mandatory root cause analysis for a serious event, it is important not to leave anything blank in the report. In other words, if the environment did not play a part in contributing to the occurrence, write that no environmental factors contributed. If you do that, then the reviewer realizes that you addressed the issue and came to a conclusion about it. If you leave the form blank, it may be that you simply don't know. There's a big difference.

It may be wise to gather a group together to write the report. For example, in the medication error example the managers of several services should be involved in the RCA and in developing improvements and monitoring procedures—certainly those responsible for education of nurses and residents, ICU nurse managers, critical care nursing unit managers, pharmacists, and physicians. Everyone involved in the incident needs to be accountable and to understand what went wrong and where the risk points exist in the process. The goal of doing the analysis of the event is to improve patient safety, to ensure that risks are minimized and that future occurrences are avoided. There is no way to accomplish this unless the information is complete.

Corrective Action

Not only are you expected to analyze an event, the regulatory agencies also require that you propose and implement a corrective action plan. As we have said, it is not enough to know what went wrong (which is often difficult enough), corrective actions have to be developed and implemented so that similar occurrences are avoided in the future. The manager is involved in all phases of the RCA, the discovery, the analysis, the development of improvements, the implementation of new processes, and the monitoring of the success of the new processes. Therefore, it is important that you involve your own manager, who needs to realize that new processes are being developed and do what is needed to support them.

Corrective actions are expected to be developed and implemented quickly but safely. Improvements can be carefully monitored and evaluated by the relevant department managers and by quality management to make certain that they do what they are supposed to do. Obviously, you can't correct a problem until you analyze what happened.

Once you develop a plan for improvement, you need to define a time line for implementation. Therefore, it has to be doable. You don't want to put a corrective action in place that would take years to implement or one that is unreasonable given the circumstances of your institution. You want to keep it realistic. And what is more important, you want to be able to measure its success so you can monitor the improvements. So make it practical, make it possible to implement within a specific—short—time frame, and make it measurable for monitoring its success. Once a new policy is developed, it is a good idea for a manager to observe it directly, to watch the process in action to see if it is working. If the improvement is impractical, the result will be noncompliance or staff will find shortcuts, which may result in danger to patients.

For example, if your corrective action involves educating the staff about a specific policy, you want to outline who will be educated, and how the productivity of the education will be evaluated. Who will be accountable for the education? What form will it take? How long will it take? What kind of format will be involved, and so on. It is not adequate to simply say "educate staff" as part of a corrective action.

Corrective actions should lead to best practices because processes should be significantly improved, and they should be reported out, through the communication structure, so that everyone understands the nature of the incident and the plan for improvement. At our system's PICG, corrective actions are discussed with the entire group. Often, recommendations that come from the multidisciplinary perspective add great value to the plan.

Establishing and reporting your corrective actions is just the beginning of the process. You have to keep monitoring their effectiveness. You won't know if the improvement is ongoing and permanent unless you track and trend over time. Again, having data makes all the difference. Once you determine an effective corrective action, collect information about the process you are correcting. Most often, the Quality Management Department at the institution will work with managers about developing and monitoring the effectiveness of the corrective action. You'll know if your corrective action is effective if the problem is not recurring, or, if the problem itself is unavoidable, fail-safe mechanisms are in place that preserve patient safety. The JCAHO recommends tracking the corrective action for six months to ensure education of all staff and effectiveness of the changes.

For example, a reasonable corrective action for the medication error example discussed earlier would be to revise the medication administration process so that it is simpler and avoids confusion regarding the correct amount of the drug as well as the route of administration. For safety and clarity of the process, the physician should have to use a special form for high-risk medications that details the dosage, calculated according to the patient's weight, and includes a time frame for administration—how long and how often. Another correction would be to prohibit the Pharmacy from sending undiluted high-risk medications to the unit and to require Pharmacy staff to prepare all intravenous infusion medications. All Nursing and Pharmacy staff should undergo education about critical care drug calculations, including dosage for both intravenous one-time infusions and drip preparation. Medical residents could be educated about medication delivery and a revised chain of command could be established to increase accountability and include a higher level of medical coverage.

Incidents can lead to changes in practices and policies. Ongoing competency assessment for house staff and ICU nurses can be conducted, including a simulated medication lab. Pharmacists should also be educated regarding drug calculation and be expected to complete a written test reflecting competency. The hospital might implement a new model for medical coverage in the ICU, with a supervising intensivist or certified critical care physician available 24/7 to provide ongoing care for patients and supervision of residents. Full-time intensivists also improve communication with nurses and other practitioners (such as respiratory therapists) providing care to these patients as long as the manager sets the appropriate expectations.

A hospital-wide multidisciplinary team can oversee the medication error reduction initiative. The nurse manager can conduct concurrent chart reviews on all critical care units to ensure appropriate preparation of all identified emergency IV drips and can use observation to ensure that appropriate techniques are in place for handling medications. All orientation and education programs should require a perfect score for passing (this is one area where you *can* insist on zero defect). Medication errors should be formally reported on a monthly basis, aggregated by Quality Management, and communicated throughout the entire continuum of care to increase every manager's awareness of the processes that produced the error and the actions taken to eliminate it.

Ensuring Success

Errors and near misses occur for many reasons, and it is important to try and come to grips with them. Errors are most often made by competent people who, for reasons that need to be understood, have performed poorly. The reasons could be personal, such as increased stress, fatigue, or distraction, or more organizational, such as the unit's being short-staffed or having inadequate policies, not enough redundancy, and so on. Usually the reason for an error involves both individual and organizational factors. We have spoken throughout this book about standardizing care and reducing variation in care. If everyone is delivering medication the same way, the right way, few if any errors would occur in the delivery of medication. Yet most health care organizations have many such errors—and more near misses. If everyone at all times followed the policies and procedures developed for operative site verification, few if any wrong site surgeries would occur. Yet there are wrong site surgeries. Working toward eliminating variation and standardizing care can help reduce errors. Constant vigilance by the manager is required to monitor and evaluate all processes on the unit.

Monitoring corrective action requires data and is as complex an endeavor as any other measurement collection and analysis. For example, processes and detailed procedures are in place for obtaining informed consent and for operative site verification (among many others). For informed consent the specific physician who is performing the procedure has to be identified. How do we know this is indeed happening across our vast system? How do we check the compliance rate? It is impractical to try and examine every single informed consent document, which means that a sample has to be examined and measurements need to be defined. Collection procedures for the data have to be identified and a reporting procedure developed. If the results reveal poor compliance, corrective action has to be planned. That action has to be measured and monitored to determine its effectiveness and then the data regarding the improvement should be communicated to the appropriate units. All this takes time. Sending a piece of paper with a corrective action to the Joint Commission after an event doesn't correct the problem. But using the PDCA methodology will.

Usually the manager will be responsible for the ongoing oversight to determine whether or not improvements are successful and staff is complying with new processes and procedures. If the manager helps educate frontline staff about the real risks involved in taking shortcuts or doing something out of convenience, fewer shortcuts will be taken. That nurse who relied on her memory might not have put the blood vial in her pocket if she had been aware that a patient could be hurt by that action. No one wants patients to be harmed. But it may require education to make sure that people realize how what seems a natural and trivial variation from the standard procedures could lead to a serious incident.

SUMMARY

The manager's role in managing errors and incidents involves the following actions:

- Make sure that patients are safe and protected from unnecessary harm.
- Constantly assess risks in the environment of care.
- Analyze process flaws discovered through RCA or FMEA that damage patient safety.
- Maintain relationships in the community.
- Proactively implement improvements in vulnerable processes.
- Establish criteria for vendors to interact with patient care.
- Determine accountability for staff.
- Develop contingency plans for potential failures in the delivery of care.
- Assess the formal and informal practices in various processes.
- Discover the barriers to effective communication and implement improvement and education to eliminate them.
- Maintain staff proficiency regarding technology dependent processes.
- Encourage a culture of teamwork around the common goal—of patient safety.
- Identify reasons that procedures fail and correct them.
- Communicate openly and honestly with patients about errors.
- Revise policies for common procedures that have risks to patients.
- Define *error* and *near miss* for the staff.
- React to small problems before they become big ones.
- Investigate the causes of an incident with an open mind.
- Use the reporting process as an opportunity to improve care.
- Require that staff provide a level of detail regarding the whys of an incident.
- Address all the issues that may have been relevant to an incident.

- Implement a corrective action plan that is realistic and measurable.
- Communicate the results of an incident analysis and correction plans across the hospital.
- Monitor improvements through data collection and analysis.

Things to Think About

- What would be a reportable incident on your service or department? Do an RCA on this incident.
- Could an FMEA have prevented this event from happening? What processes would have been identified as flaws?

CHAPTER TEN

Working Together

When an organization is committed to quality and safety and supports a pervasive quality management structure, various elements, processes, and services become connected, like individual bricks bound together by mortar to create a single strong edifice. Quality management functions as a great equalizer because its methodology is grounded in data, and data are neutral; no single piece of information has more or less power or prestige than another. If you are lucky enough to work in a health system where quality care is integral to the mission and vision of the organization, quality management will be incorporated into every level and across all levels of the institution and the system. Keeping the patient as the focal point of analyses and gathering data regarding the delivery of care and services to the patient requires that communication among departments and among levels within departments is free flowing and accessible.

CROSSING BOUNDARIES

Quality information, to be useful, must cross all organizational boundaries and travel freely through the entire table of organization.

Traditionally, in most health care departments, staff reports to a department manager or supervisor who in turn reports to a senior or division manager who reports eventually to a vice president who reports to a senior vice president who reports to the CEO. Information moves vertically within departments, traveling up and down this hierarchy. However, a strong quality management structure requires mutual cooperation, where everyone's information is valued equally and where communication flows laterally, diagonally, and in every direction.

In addition to crossing departmental and service lines, quality management also interacts with all levels of administration because everyone has a common goal: to provide good outcomes. If outcomes are good and the resulting data support the claim that the hospital is delivering a quality product in the form of excellent care, patients return, and administrative goals are achieved. More and more administrators, from individual department heads up the hierarchy to the highest levels of the organization, are beginning to use quality data to monitor care services and evaluate providers and departments.

Uniting Services

In our health care system, the CEO meets weekly with senior staff from various departments and reviews a set of quality indicators that illuminates information about care in the different hospitals and across the system. The information can be compared to the dashboard of a car, where at a single glance the driver can view the various gauges that reflect the workings of critical systems and know if some area requires attention or repair or if all is well (see Figure 10.1).

The dashboard report further confirms the interconnectedness of all services because information, in the form of indicators, is displayed and discussed as representing a single endeavor—providing patients with quality care—rather than reports from individual departments.

Figure 10.2 is an example of the format in which we report measures to senior leadership. The process of evaluating the delivery of care via the quality indicators for all services must be ongoing and frequent in order to be effective. At the weekly meetings of the senior staff, aggregated data for the quarter is compared with past quarters to track and trend improvements. By displaying and discussing information relevant to each hospital and the entire system and by meeting together to evaluate the information, sharing and communicating critical data across service lines, the senior staff functions as a team.

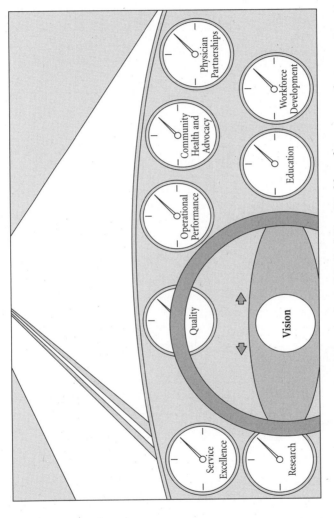

Figure 10.1.   Medical Care Dashboard.

Indicators
Case Mix Index
Overall Excess Days
Inlier Excess Days
Outlier Excess Days
Rate of Unplanned Readmissions to Hospital Within 30 Days
Rate of Med/Surg Nosocomial Pressure Ulcer
Medication Error Rate
Mortality Case Mix Index
Surgical Site Infection Rate
Clinical Pathway – Congestive Heart Failure
• Rate of Patients Discharged on Clinical Pathway 311
• Rate of Patients Discharged on Triple (Diuretic, Digoxin, & ACEI) Therapy
• Rate of Patients Who Received Nutritional Counseling
Clinical Pathway – Simple Pneumonia
• Rate of Patients Discharged on Clinical Pathway 330
• Rate of Patients Switched to Oral Antibiotics on Day 4
Core Measures – Heart Failure
• Rate of Patients with LVF Evaluation Before, During or Planned D/C
Core Measures – Simple Pneumonia
• Time (mean mins.) to Antibiotic
Core Measures – AMI
• Rate of Patients Who Received ASA 24 Hours Before or After Arrival
Rate of Unplanned Returns to OR Within 30 days
Rate of Unplanned Extubation (*ICU only*)
ICU Crude Mortality
Indexes
Fall Index
Adult Med/Surg Restraint Episode Index
LWOBE Index
Return Within 72 Hours of ED Discharge Index

Figure 10.2.   Table of Measures Format.

Year 2002	Q1 2002	Q2 2002	Q3 2002	Q4 2002

So often in health care institutions, the right hand doesn't know what the left hand is doing because so little communication passes between departments or services. When the organization creates a structure where information is shared and communication is mandatory, divisions and separations begin to merge and blend.

Multidisciplinary Performance Improvement

Because the senior leaders are genuinely dedicated to working together to improve performance, the staff they supervise are comfortable reflecting their values and thus are willing to share information across disciplines as well. This is seen most clearly through the authentically democratic and multidisciplinary PICGs that monitor the delivery of care for each hospital and for the health system. Improvement initiatives have succeeded in large part because these groups encourage individuals from different services to come together, bringing with them their specialized expertise, to review issues and make suggestions. Their meetings are conducted in a climate of respect and tolerance for the views held by others. When improvements are developed and implemented, they quickly earn a broad range of professional buy-in, since diverse input has been considered and included.

The PICGs provide a forum for people who rarely have the opportunity to talk to each other or to have their views heard. For example, in the normal course of the workday housekeeping staff may have little occasion to interact with laboratory technicians; nutritionists might not have much contact with engineers; and ancillary professionals such as respiratory therapists rarely mingle with members of the Finance Department. Through the holistic view of the delivery of health care services, as supported by the PICGs, it becomes increasingly obvious that everyone has much to learn about how much each service depends on other services. No department can function independently to deliver quality care—and shouldn't even try. Figure 10.3 depicts the many departments that interact within the PICG framework.

Managing to Communicate

Each of the different hospitals that make up the NS-LIJHS, whether one of the tertiary teaching hospitals or the smaller community hospitals, has formed its own multidisciplinary PICG. In the administrative offices of the health system, representatives from the eighteen

hospitals meet at a system-level PICG to discuss and review performance issues and to recommend and monitor improvement efforts. We
have found that once people from different areas within the hospital
and from different hospitals start talking to each other, the benefits—
personal, organizational, and for the patient—are enormous.

In addition, our PICG meetings introduce middle management directly into the conversation about prioritized improvement efforts. As
those who are most familiar with the actual daily activities of their departments, close to the frontline workers, and with access to the higher-
level managers who make policy decisions, managers can provide input
crucial to understanding both the care that is being delivered and any
of the problems involved in delivering that care, problems that lead to
the kinds of shortcuts and creative adaptations that were discussed in
Chapter Nine.

Exchanging ideas within the forum of the PICG has the further advantage of reducing the isolation of the managers and illustrating to
them how their work fits into the context of a patient's hospital
episode. If managers are isolated in their own units, as they so often
are, they naturally find it difficult to understand the import of certain
defined goals. For example, if you manage a Housekeeping service,
and you design bed turnover processes without knowing the expectations of the nurses on the unit, you will be hard-pressed to conform
your goals to theirs.

But if you are cognizant of the fact that a quick bed turnover will
reduce bottlenecks in the ED because patients will be more speedily
transferred to the units and new patients will be efficiently admitted
to the units, your process becomes sensible in terms of the larger picture. Furthermore, as your staff comes to recognize the ramifications
of their responsibility and work with the nurses on the unit to provide for the next admission speedily, the patient and the organization
become increasingly well served.

Keep the Conversation Going

The exchange of information and communication cannot be sporadic;
to be effective it must exist within organized and well-established
channels. The PICGs in each hospital and at the system level meet
monthly, with special subcommittees, charged with developing new
processes or analyzing procedures for possible improvement, that meet
more frequently as needed.

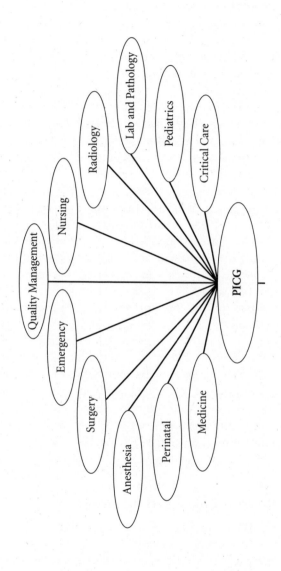

Committees (*Monthly Report*)

Blood (Transfusion Committee)	Patient Safety
Credentialing	Pharmacy and Therapeutics
Ethics	Radiation Safety
Health Information Management	Safety
Infection Control	Tissue

Support Functions (*Quarterly Report*)

Ambulatory Care	Finance and Admitting	Physical Therapy
Discharge Planning	Food and Nutrition	Respiratory Therapy
Education and Training	Human Resources	Risk Management
Engineering	Materials Management	Social Work
Environmental Services	Patient Issues and Patient Satisfaction	Utilization Management

Figure 10.3.   Hospital Performance Improvement Coordinating Group.

The monthly meetings keep communication continual and quality expectations high. Constant dialogue, which might otherwise not exist, links the various departments. Since managers are primarily responsible for coordinating improvement activities, their involvement at these meetings is expected and welcomed, and their input is crucial. The PICGs help to prioritize improvements and develop plans for them. Even more important, they monitor and evaluate the effectiveness of the improvement efforts through measurements that are presented to the committee on an ongoing basis. All these activities require the very active engagement of the managers.

In addition to the hospital PICG structure, the hundreds of ambulatory sites associated with the health system have coordinated their care through forming and participating in their own system Ambulatory PICG so that common concerns are discussed and improvements standardized. For example, if immunization of two-year-olds or flu shots for adults, defined as part of the national agenda for patient safety, is not being measured, success or failure cannot be tracked and monitored. Through the structure of the ambulatory PICGs, definitions were determined for measurement; the administrative managers of the ambulatory sites received welcome tools to track patient volume and compliance rates, and were thus able to target areas for improvement.

Rather than functioning outside the core of the system like neglected stepchildren, quality management processes have brought the ambulatory practices into the loop of coordinated care. For example, information about Pap smear rates (testing for cervical cancer) is tracked across the sites. Depending on the result of the test, patients may need the services of the laboratory or the Pharmacy, and may require follow-up care by the Ambulatory Practice physician, or even need input from Social Work. Without the quality measurement methodology coordinating information, the system would not be able to track and treat patients from diagnosis to discharge.

The JCAHO recognizes that unless the patient experience is coherent from admission to discharge, the system risks breaches in the care the patient receives. To avoid this, it is essential to review how the patient moves through the continuum of care. Many health care institutions do not have a single organizing structure that monitors and evaluates the safety of patients throughout their involvement with the system; a strong quality management communication structure provides this function. If there is a break in the delivery of care, the patient usually suffers and the cost to the institution goes up.

Not only is superior communication good for the patient, it is also good business. The PICG structure far surpasses the expectations of the JCAHO, which simply requires that an organization monitor its performance; the agency does not dictate how this should be accomplished or what level of sophistication is expected. Further, the JCAHO does not evaluate the results of improvement efforts; that is left to the hospital to do.

Coordinating Services

Before managers can meaningfully participate in a hospital-wide discussion of quality, however, they have to be able to articulate their scope of care, delineate the function of their department, and quantify that care so it is readily understood by individuals from other departments. You should be able to explain the specific goals of your patient population and define how these goals are accomplished. Physical Therapy, for example, might define its goal as improving the range and motion of the patient, or Engineering might define its goal as maintaining proper airflow and temperature in the operating rooms.

Further, managers should be able to specify the target of their service. Physical Therapy may define orthopedic patients, stroke patients, the elderly, or women recovering from mastectomy as appropriate recipients of services. Identifying the patient population includes understanding the distinct and specific requirements that have to be analyzed and understood before care can be delivered efficiently.

Another consideration in defining the scope of care and how your service interacts with other services in managing the patient involves determining under what circumstances you deliver your care to your specific population. If Physical Therapy works with orthopedic patients after surgery with the goal of increasing motion and does not establish communication with the clinical staff caring for the patient, therapists may not realize that their work can reduce clotting or decrease pain. They may not recognize cases where it would be useful to involve Social Work. However, if they understand the relationship between their goals and the clinical import of their service, care for the patient is better integrated and improved.

If the range of motion for a mastectomy patient increases, perhaps that improvement has an impact on pain and on depression, both of which may influence patient satisfaction, discharge date, and LOS. Physical Therapy can improve care for the elderly by working with

Nursing on the floors to educate nurses about how to take a patient out of bed safely, thereby increasing mobility for the patient and improving quality of life.

It is not unusual for Engineering staff to do their job without understanding the clinical implications of maintaining the equipment. But through quality, a dialogue between Nursing and Engineering occurs, with information shared about the role of IV pumps or OR airflow in maintaining health or reducing infection. As an engineer, if you understand the relationship between temperature and infection, it puts your work into a larger context and gives you the information you need to understand risk to the patient. Also, you will be better prepared to do critical thinking during a disruption of normal routines such as occurs when an incident happens.

Working with the PICG committees allows engineers to interact with the rest of the hospital community and so work in a more integrated environment. Rather than simply conforming to a requirement that the airflow in the OR should be this or that, for example, the engineer grasps the critical interaction between airflow and infection. Such an understanding might increase the Engineering Department's desire to develop quality control mechanisms and indicators as well as to outline a timetable for preventive maintenance of equipment.

In other words, if you define your job as you might in a job description, without understanding the complex interactions and interrelationships among services and with the ultimate goal of improving patient well-being, then you don't understand your role and will find it difficult to contribute to the organization's goals. But if you can outline your scope of care in the terms suggested here, your contribution to understanding clinical care and to performance improvement will be more valuable.

DOING THE RIGHT THING WELL TOGETHER

Although specific services and disciplines define their own values for what a good outcome entails, an outcome is actually the end result of many people collaborating together in complex processes. Good outcomes are determined by your priorities within your special scope of care and your philosophy or vision of the kind of care you want to deliver. Your actions or interventions—or lack of them—lead to outcomes. If your interventions are good, the outcome is likely to be good.

Managers should monitor the activities of each day. Review your patient population and their diagnoses and treatment plans. If you identify or suspect any weak areas, communicate to your staff to prevent any interruption to a proper flow of patients through the unit or the services delivered to the patient. Visit each patient to assure yourself about the standard of care being delivered and that your unit is meeting the patient's expectations. Such an approach will result in good outcomes.

Managing Outcomes

The managers set the definition for what a good outcome would be on their services and train staff accordingly. If your definition of a good outcome is to provide good skin care, for example, then you can monitor the incidence and severity of skin ulcers on your unit—and if data reveal that the care requires improvement, you can introduce new processes or enhance education for your staff. If you are responsible for bed turnover, you monitor turnaround time and assess if it is improving and if you are reaching your own predetermined goals. If so, then you are providing a good outcome on your service. If you manage a Radiology unit, your definition of a good outcome might be not repeating films, or making sure that patients are appropriately screened for X-rays and other technology.

More and more government agencies such as the CMS, or national monitoring groups such as the AHCPR, PROs, and the National Patient Safety Foundation, use outcomes to assess the effectiveness of medical interventions and to evaluate under- and overuse of services that are reflected in cost. Subjective data, such as quality of life or emotional status reports, have been added to the more traditional outcomes of mortality, readmissions, and complications.

Outcomes assessment may be an effective barometer for patients to understand and evaluate their care as well, and may serve to improve education and decision making regarding choices related to that care. If patients on your unit with CHF are not educated regarding the importance of monitoring their weight, that is not a good outcome because weight management and nutritional education are paramount to the success of treatment. Or if you are managing a Patient Relations division and it is your job to ensure that visitors don't get lost, and Reception is always crowded and long lines back up in front of information counters, that is not a good outcome. If you make changes, put up signs and maps, stagger visiting hours, or implement other improvements targeted at improving congestion, and if such interventions are effective according to the patient satisfaction data that you collect, then you have better outcomes. Good management often involves taking a proactive approach to the services you deliver and introducing improvements before you have problems to correct.

As manager, you are accountable to your manager and administration for providing your patients with good outcomes. You can't do this alone, and so you need the respect and confidence of your staff. If people who work for you feel you are encouraging them to grow professionally and to take an active role in the delivery of care, and that you trust them to do the right thing the right way at the right time, they will respond with enthusiasm. When people see they are valued, they do the best job possible. You set the bar for your staff.

You accomplish this by defining your values and transmitting them to your staff. If a patient complains that a nurse had to try several times before successfully drawing blood, and you respond by saying that such events occur only a small percentage of the time, that sends a signal about your expectations to your staff. You don't expect 100 percent. Is that the message you want to send? You and the administration of your hospital put a value on the services delivered, and those values establish expectations for the provision of care, which leads to good or bad outcomes for the patient.

If you are responsible for the housekeeping on a unit, you might expect it to have adequate lighting at night. Your goal is to provide a safe and comfortable environment for the patient. If the lights are on, that is a good outcome, as you have defined it. If a light is out, is a process in place for replacing it in a timely way? Who is accountable? If it matters to you as a manager, then it will matter to your staff. If not, not. This seems a small matter, but it is symbolic of the details of care you deliver. If you were at home, you would not want to walk around in the dark because the lightbulbs were burned out. Do you treat your patients as you would your family, or do you make assumptions that the details of your patients' comfort are different from your own? Florence Nightingale thought no detail too small, and set expectations for airflow and cleanliness, lighting and privacy. Her expectations were very high and very precise. Are yours?

Maintain Vigilance

In addition to setting expectations regarding outcomes for your staff, you need to monitor the delivery of care on a continuous basis. One good outcome does not predict that good outcomes will occur all the time. Unfortunately, it is very easy for people to become complacent with routines, and complacency can lead to inadequate care and thus poor outcomes. If your staff knows you are vigilant, they will be too. Many managers are so overloaded with work that they spend their time plugging up deficits in care that erupt into crises, an effort that leaves little time or energy for adequate management. Leadership—and a manager is the leader of the service or unit—should be more than that. Complacency and overwork can easily lead to a poor outcome, or even an incident.

As we have said, an outcome is the result of the work of many people. Think of an operating room. It is a high-risk environment because of the vulnerability of surgical patients and the possibility for infection, which has been identified by the IOM as a preventable cause of hospital death. Many individuals are responsible for maintaining the sterile integrity of the OR: the room must be cleaned between procedures and at the end of the day; airflow and ventilation should be monitored on an ongoing basis; the equipment must be sterilized and stored appropriately. All personnel must know and follow detailed policies and procedures.

Now imagine the following scenario: A surgeon is performing an operation and everything is going well. Suddenly water starts leaking from the ceiling onto the patient. As OR manager, what would be your immediate response—regarding the environment of the OR, toward the patient, and to the administration? How would you address this situation? You could panic and run around and be worried about a lawsuit, or you could transfer the patient at once to another OR, ensure that the patient is safe, close the compromised OR, contact Engineering, and discover why the problem occurred. Could it have been prevented, and if so, were adequate preventive measures in place and being monitored? Who is accountable?

To successfully conduct an investigation into the causes of this incident, the OR manager would have to communicate with the Engineering Department and the managers there, and be working perhaps with Housekeeping, Safety, and Infection Control, and with physicians and nursing staff as well as Risk Management and the administration. The manager should conduct an RCA with individuals from the relevant departments to determine whether the cause of the problem was an unavoidable random accident or a symptom of an ongoing problem that requires correction.

Several lessons can be learned from this example. All employees, including the support staff, are responsible for the success of a procedure or the lack of it. All environments should be checked by the manager and staff just as pilots assess their planes before take-off. Simply because everything was working smoothly one day does not guarantee that all will be well the next. Don't relax your vigilance, and encourage your staff to be alert to the possibilities of flaws in the system as well. Use the technique of FMEA for high-risk processes to identify risk points for the patient.

Once the patient is transferred and safe, other issues still require management. An empty OR makes a terrific dent in a hospital's budget, a consideration that may deter some managers from closing it. Should you reopen the OR after putting a pail down to collect water, or do you need to shut down the room, and perhaps all the other ORs as well, until you understand the full scope of the problem? Why did this particular event happen at this time? Perhaps if the Engineering manager had done a better job of preventive maintenance and been on top of the situation, the event might not have occurred, and patient safety might have been preserved. As you can see, not doing the right thing on a continuous basis can lead to enormous expense. Once you understand what happened and why and what risk points require monitoring to prevent similar occurrences, you will be able to make informed and intelligent decisions about how to manage your service.

Managing Clinical Care

Another opportunity for the manager to coordinate care and interact with the clinical staff is in the development of policies and procedures. Managers' opinions regarding quality are sought out and valued by medical boards, especially to determine if and how the standard of care can be achieved. When you are able to define the scope of care as well as the goals for your patients, and you understand the relationship between the service you are responsible for and its interconnections with other services and disciplines, you can productively discuss patient care with physicians and can help physicians understand the problems and concerns of the frontline workers involved in delivering that care.

The medical board sets the standard of care, and determines, for example, that pneumonia patients should have antibiotics administered within four hours of admission. Such a standard affects Pharmacy and Nursing staff, as well as the unit managers. The managers can inform the physician if they encounter roadblocks to delivering this service, and perhaps have some realistic ideas for improvements.

When our health system was working to formulate guidelines for bariatric surgery, many different departments participated in the discussion, and therefore the input of many managers was solicited. Nutritionists, psychologists, and social workers were involved because they are critical to the initial evaluation and assessment of the patient. Medicine, Nursing, Anesthesia, and ICU managers were also consulted. Engineering and Materials Support Services were brought into the meetings because specialized equipment is necessary to ensure safety of the obese patients undergoing this surgery.

Through the quality management committee structure, staff came together to develop and implement standards of care. But the work doesn't stop there. Once developed and implemented, the care must be monitored over time, measurements must be defined, and data must be collected, analyzed, interpreted, and reported back to the relevant disciplines. The results of the data collection over time must be reviewed on an ongoing basis to ensure that the standards are in fact being met.

The PDCA methodology promotes continuing dialogue among managers and other caregivers regarding procedures. The Plan phase to develop guidelines for bariatric surgery involved months of discussion among disciplines to brainstorm issues and to reach consensus regarding appropriate and reasonable protocols. The time was well spent, because the discussions permitted caregivers from various disciplines to interact and to learn about one another's concerns.

The Do phase involved defining the qualifications for the surgeon who would perform this risky procedure as well as the criteria for patients who would be appropriate to receive it. It was important to determine the departments that would be involved with the patient in preparation for the procedure; therefore managers of Social Work, Nutrition, Psychology, Internal Medicine, Surgery, and Nursing were included in these discussions. Postoperative care and monitoring the patient after hospitalization also required definition.

As part of the Check phase, measures were defined that would evaluate the quality of care delivered, such as reoperation, rehospitalization within thirty days, quality of life (for example, depression), wound infection, weight gain or loss, and complications or mortality within thirty days of the procedure. In the Act phase, the protocols were implemented and evaluated through the measurements. Best practices were defined.

In institutions with weak Quality Management Departments and minimal leadership commitment to quality, managers frequently have few opportunities to express their opinions, to interact with policy-makers, or to expose their concerns and problems. They work alone, supervising their own staff and wrestling with their own problems in relative isolation. However, with a strong Quality Management Department, communication with the manager is actively sought. When a new procedure such as bariatric surgery is being developed, it is the frontline manager who is asked to educate the medical boards on the practicality of the particulars of the procedure in the existing working environment. If changes need to be made to implement new procedures so that they will be more effective, it is the manager who can outline what those changes should be.

Furthermore, it is the manager who will monitor the new procedure, oversee the new protocols, and report back through the committee structure if any problems occur. It is the manager who understands the competency requirements of the staff involved and can communicate in both directions, to the medical boards and to the bedside staff, if in-service or any other education is necessary to successfully implement the new program.

The Leadership Connection

The quality management structure at the NS-LIJHS system involves the managers at an even higher level, that of the Board of Trustees. The Joint Conference Professional Affairs Committees (JCPACs) were created expressly to further communication between the highest levels of the organization and the daily workers. Often, in a complex organization, the bureaucracy and red tape involved in moving information among different parts of the institution hinder communication. The different JCPAC committees were designed expressly to facilitate multidisciplinary input in order to fulfill their charge to prioritize areas for evaluation and improvement.

For example, Quality Management investigated issues relating to the care of patients with sleep apnea, a relatively common condition that restricts airflow. To safeguard hospitalized patients with sleep apnea, especially those who require anesthesia for surgery, a performance improvement initiative was presented to the JCPAC for Acute Care. Anesthesia collaborated with Pulmonary Medicine, Surgery, Respiratory Care, and the intensivists and nurses involved in presurgical assessment, perioperative nursing, and postoperative care to develop guidelines for how best to administer anesthesia and care of this patient population. The JCPAC suggested a systemwide acceptance of these guidelines, which were then brought back to each hospital's medical board for approval.

Because the success of an improvement effort such as this must involve various managers, managers were invited to participate in these meetings and express their opinions about issues related to the delivery of care. Such interactions enhance accountability for everyone involved. To interact with the governing body, the manager has to be well versed not only on the scope of care, the goal of the care being delivered, and how the manager's service interacts with others in the hospital but also in areas of quality, such as measurements, assessment, monitoring, and evaluation tools—all the methodology associated with performance improvement. Managers prepared in this way are in a position to intelligently inform the Board about their concerns.

In many health care systems managers do not have a chance to express themselves either in front of their peers or before the leaders of their organizations. We have found that a strong quality management infrastructure, one that defines goals for patients and is acknowledged by all, recognizes the contribution of all the employees within the system with the respect they deserve. Just as in industry, where those businesses whose workers own stock and have a vested interest in the company's success are more productive, financially stable, and have greater employee satisfaction, in health care it is simply good business to involve the daily worker in the common goal of preserving patient safety and delivering quality services.

Another place where the department head, supervisor, or manager has an opportunity to interact with members of the Board and senior leadership is during the executive session, a forum expressly designed to allow sensitive information to be shared, discussed, and acted upon while preserving privacy and confidentiality. During the executive session of the Board, when adverse or serious incidents are discussed, managers are often called upon to explain to leadership not only what happened and why but also what corrective actions were taken, what monitoring systems were developed to prevent a repeat event, what educational measures were implemented, and what best practices have been established.

Managing Information

Without a working familiarity with quality management tools, a manager would be hard-pressed to provide these committees with the information they require. Since the analyses of adverse events require representation from many departments and disciplines, defining and understanding important issues affecting patient safety must be the responsibility of many managers, who are expected to function as an integrated team. The respect of the leadership for this process reinforces to the managers that they are considered professionals whose insight into the processes of care is necessary for performance improvement.

The members of the Board and senior leadership, having been educated in quality management methodology, are able to use quality management data to evaluate and review any deviation in care within the hospital or system and make recommendations for improvements. Familiarity with quality management techniques thus helps each manager inform the leadership about how to improve care. If one hospital has shown success in a specific area of patient care, the Board may recommend that the best practices from that hospital or unit be tried in another hospital. Therefore, managers at one hospital are expected to interact with managers from others throughout the system to develop and implement best practices.

Since mistakes are inevitable and no one can control every aspect of care delivery, it is expected that all managers will have to face a crisis at some time. Such an event needs to be reported to the regulatory agencies and to the governing board. In addition, an accrediting body may find some aspect of the delivery of care that should be improved to maintain patient safety. The manager who is familiar with quality methods such as RCA and FMEA can communicate more effectively about gaps in the delivery of care and be precise and explicit about how to develop preventive action. The role of manager becomes highly visible when working within a quality management structure and communicating vertically and horizontally across the organization. Staff like to follow a leader who knows what to do, when to do it, and how to talk about it intelligently.

ON COMMON GROUND

Many departments work closely with the Quality Management Department and become incorporated into the quality infrastructure because goals for patient care and organizational performance are intertwined. The more education regarding quality processes that managers possess, the better able they are to integrate improvement efforts.

The following examples of collaboration among departments illustrate how valuable it is to work together to achieve a common goal.

Quality and Risk Management

Many health systems combine Risk Management and the Quality Management Department. In our system, the two departments are separate, but they work very closely together. The goals of both departments are congruent. One of the goals for Risk Management is to anticipate potential malpractice claims and make every effort to reduce them. One of the goals of Quality Management is to prevent the kinds of problems that result in malpractice claims. Obviously, they share a common agenda, since preventing adverse occurrences reduces malpractice claims. Prevention up front reduces incidents. Using quality management tools such as the RCA and FMEA, statistics, and databases, especially about adverse events, the two departments share information and communicate about improvement efforts.

If Risk Management has a cluster of claims regarding certain types of injuries—for example, Erb's Palsy, a pediatric condition that had been associated with problems incurred during labor and delivery—the Quality Management Department can provide information about causality: What are the benchmarks nationally for Erb's Palsy? How frequently does it occur? What kinds of delivery issues are related to it, if any, and what are any general risk factors associated with its occurrence, either in the pregnancy or with delivery? Once the causality is analyzed, programs can be developed, through the quality management structure, to improve education for physicians and nurses regarding safeguards and risks for this condition. The manager monitors and evaluates the improvements.

When our health system analyzed the incidence and risks associated with Erb's Palsy, we used statistical data to educate caregivers and implement programs that resulted in reducing its incidence. Once that occurred, Risk Management negotiated with our insurance company for a reduced premium on the basis that we could illustrate that the event was no longer a completely random happening but one about which we had a great deal of information and had implemented improvement efforts. As a result of the collaboration between Risk Management and Quality Management and with medical and Nursing staff, patient safety was improved and costs were reduced. Everyone benefits when departments work together.

Quality Management and Finance

Quality Management and the Finance Department also work hand in hand to mutual advantage and to the benefit of the patients and the health system. One of the goals of the Finance Department is to ensure that appropriate reimbursement is made for services rendered, which depends on the accurate coding of services and thorough documentation in the medical record. Documentation is also required by the Quality Management Department to collect the information necessary for the development of measurements to monitor and improve outcomes.

Both Quality Management and Finance scrutinize resources to ensure that patients are using clinical services appropriately. Overutilization of services is not only bad for the patient, it results in increased costs to the hospital. Underutilization is also not beneficial for the patient and may result in complications and readmission that require long LOS. Managed care has forced further collaboration between Quality Management and Finance in the analysis of denials, which must be monitored and evaluated carefully or the cost to the institution could be very high.

Financial information depends, in part, on physician orders for services, and those orders are incorporated into the guidelines established through the quality management structure. Guidelines help ensure that care is appropriate, and using guidelines not only promotes good care but has the advantage of regulating documentation through guideline variance forms. Monitoring LOS and collecting data regarding services and LOS helps both departments understand utilization and where improvement efforts should be directed. Every manager has to be responsive to budgetary concerns, which are greatly influenced by utilization of services, efficiencies, and good quality outcomes.

Quality Management and Materials Support Services

Materials Support Services (MSS) also works closely with Quality Management, drawing on quality data to understand the clinical need for materials such as specialty beds, medications, and other resources. Historically MSS based its decisions about what to order on past use. Faced with a change in pattern, such as an upsurge of the need for a piece of equipment, MSS could encounter delays in supplying what was necessary.

Using the quality management database helps MSS make purchasing decisions based on a more clinical approach. For example, when the database showed a steady decline in decubiti across the system, MSS had a rationale for ordering fewer specialty beds. After several years the collaboration between the two departments led to an economic partnership between our institution and the specialty bed rental company, creating further efficiencies that reduced costs.

The quality management database also permitted MSS to streamline and standardize the drug formulary across the system, again improving cost-effectiveness. The relationship between the two departments helps MSS be more responsive to budget constraints. When leadership asks why certain equipment was ordered or why so many identical items were requested, or why some equipment or medication needed to be replaced, or why it wasn't replaced, quality data make it feasible to provide these answers.

By participating in the PICG meetings, MSS managers develop a level of comfort that they understand the entire process and know how and where their materials fit into providing quality care across the continuum. For example, Quality Management and Materials Support Services collaborated on a sterilization improvement effort for the operating room that began by taking an inventory of the different sterilization tools and procedures used across the system. The goal was to reduce infection, make care safer, create efficiencies for appropriate utilization, and improve competency for sterilization techniques.

It wasn't clear at the outset of the initiative if infection was related to staff education or to materials and equipment. Quality indicators regarding sterilization and infection data provided information that could be trended and analyzed. As a result of the collaborative effort, sterilization equipment has been standardized across the health system. Coupled with increased competency of staff in proper use of the equipment, this measure has reduced the infection rate. Again, working together helps departments understand their pivotal role in the total delivery of care.

Quality and Emergency Services

Emergency Medical Services (EMS) staff began to monitor their delivery of care based on the quality management model. Their performance improved considerably once they collected and analyzed what they determined to be the quality indicators for their service. For example, they analyzed the amount of time it took to transport a critically ill patient from a community hospital to a tertiary facility for care. With improved education for staff and better procedures for documentation, EMS was able to significantly reduce transport time; it also introduced ICU equipment directly into the mobile units.

When EMS staff analyzed their scope of service and their patient population, they realized that a large proportion was going to the heart catheterization lab. Communicating this data through the PICG resulted in improving processes to provide a smooth transition of critically ill patients from the ED to the Cardiac Catheterization Unit. Once EMS data collection efforts had documented the volume of usage, another hospital within the system decided to build a cath lab to satisfy the excess demand the EMS reports revealed.

Through EMS quality indicators such as pediatric medication administration, patient status change en route, response times per call type, critical care transports, and cardiac arrest management, EMS determined that many transports required advanced lifesaving skills, and therefore determined to upgrade staff training so that advanced skill was available to a greater percentage of EMS staff. By introducing quality management methodology to EMS and bringing the EMS Department into the quality committee structure and including its staff in discussions regarding care across the continuum, the system is better able to serve the needs of patients in the community.

This example, like its predecessors, reflects the importance of unbiased, objective data and methodology in developing programs for providing excellent care. Collaboration among disciplines and services improves the quality of the care to the patients and the functioning of the institution.

SUMMARY

Working collaboratively in a quality management structure can help the manager manage because of the following factors:

- Quality information necessary for monitoring and improving care crosses departments and disciplines.
- Clinical and administrative leadership rely on managers for quality information about the delivery of care.

- The performance improvement coordinating groups share information across departmental lines and provide a forum for managers to express their concerns about how care is delivered.
- Information regarding the practicality of new procedures is solicited by various performance improvement groups.
- Collaboration provides a mechanism for understanding the interconnectedness of care across the continuum.
- It is easier to understand the clinical importance of each service and its responsibilities.
- Positive outcomes are the result of multidisciplinary processes.
- The staff is willing to share information for performance improvement.
- Maintaining a safe environment involves many disciplines and departments and has an impact on the budget.
- The safety of the patient across the continuum is maintained.
- Managers interact with policymakers, help patients make informed decisions, and supervise staff to improve communication among departments.
- Managers are asked by senior leadership to explain incidents and to work together to make corrective actions.

Things to Think About

- What departments and services do you interact with to manage your department or service? How do you evaluate the effectiveness of the collaboration?
- Describe a performance improvement project that would require interdepartmental collaboration.

    What data would be collected?

    How would that data be evaluated?

    Who would be primarily accountable for the improvement effort, from which service, and what would be the rationale?

Conclusion

ost managers become managers because their experience, talent, and commitment to quality care are notable. However, very few managers have the opportunity to get a training course in how to do their jobs, and fewer still enroll in an academic degree program that teaches them practical managerial skills. Throughout this book, we have tried to provide information that would give the manager, supervisor, or department head the tools and techniques necessary to become excellent at the managerial job. We have defined the role and function of the manager as an outcome-oriented position and have stressed that the goal of delivering health care services is to improve patient care with an awareness of the intricate interrelationship that exists among services.

Through the use of quality management tools and methods, managers gain an understanding of how their role fits into the larger organization and how objective data should be used to evaluate care and set clinical and utilization expectations for their department or service. Quality management methods convey a structure for introducing positive change into the delivery of care. When personal appeals have no impact, quality data, being objective and unbiased, can influence people and encourage change. Also, data can inform everyone involved in the process of care—physicians, nurses, other caregivers, and administration—about the quality of care being delivered and where opportunities for improvement exist.

Information that is gathered and analyzed through the quality management process is absolutely essential to the manager who is accountable for managing services and for improving them. Using data and quality management methodology, the manager has the opportunity to present information in its most digestible format to others and to suggest improvements based on and supported by that data. This promotes informed and balanced decision making about using resources for improving care.

Quality information also endows the manager with the leverage necessary to convince others to examine the delivery of health care services for risks to patient safety and to develop improved processes and procedures to minimize the effects of flaws in the system. Such information is crucial to hospital administrators so that they are not surprised or caught off guard by gaps in the delivery of good services. Quality information regarding the standard of care and aggregated and comparative data are critical to physicians as well, enabling them to make informed decisions regarding the best care for their patients.

On an institutional level, familiarity with quality management methodologies is essential to permit managers to operationalize and comply with regulatory issues. JCAHO standards, for example, require that leadership and staff document not only what is actually accomplished in the daily delivery of health care services but also how well it is done, which means that the managers are all expected to supply the data that evaluate the care delivered on their watch. State agencies assume that managers are familiar with the analytic processes of quality management, such as root cause analysis and failure mode effects analysis, to ensure that incidents and adverse events are properly understood and corrected. A thorough grasp of the intricacies of interrelated care that quality management allows them to monitor through indicators gives the managers a handle with which to provide efficient utilization of services. In short, to evaluate the services delivered, define weaknesses in that service, and develop improvements, managers benefit from knowing quality management methods.

Evaluating the care delivered on a unit or service requires an analysis and understanding of the outcomes or consequences of that care. Generally, it is simplistic to assume a one-to-one correspondence between quality and outcomes because sometimes the quality of care can be excellent, and yet the patient has adverse complications or a poor outcome. However, it is reasonable to infer that good outcomes are the result of quality care. The "consumer goods" that the manager is responsible for delivering and communicating are the result of the interaction between the caregiver and the patient, and the coordination of multiple services and technology that should lead to the best outcomes. Since the manager's job includes communicating to various caregivers, to the patient, the family, and the administration about patient outcomes, it is critical that the relationship between care and outcome be understood.

Defining good outcomes is also meaningful to the institution, and setting department goals and reasonable objectives that conform to the expectations established in the hospital's strategic plan is part of each manager's responsibility. For example, staffing is a constant budget item and a quality item as well. To understand the relationship between staffing and patient outcomes, the JCAHO has developed a concept that it calls "staffing effectiveness." Institutions are being asked to assess if their staffing is sufficient in numbers and competent in training to provide the expected care. The administration looks to the managers to supply information about staffing effectiveness.

How can you determine if your numbers are sufficient and that the levels of competency of your staff are adequate? If you monitor the care you deliver, collecting information on defined indicators relevant to your service, you can track the care. If there are no complaints, if there are no adverse events, if there are no falls or decubiti, and so on, can you say you have staffing effectiveness? Although you might be tempted to conclude that you do, many others factors must also be considered. Has the patient population remained constant? Perhaps there are fewer patients on the unit. (Nobody complains in an empty bed.) Is the level of competency of the staff consistent? Good care involves the interaction of many factors. Moreover, because you have been schooled in quality management methodologies, you are aware of the potential problems involved in collecting data accurately and consistently, and you can train your staff to ensure that you are interpreting reliable data. It is impossible to assess whether patient outcomes are good or poor unless you collect data. The data will also help leadership understand the relationship between staffing, for example, and patient outcomes, to better manage the budget.

To successfully balance budgetary, quality care, and patient safety concerns with outcomes, managers must learn to expertly juggle every aspect related to the delivery of care for their assigned patients. The best way to do this is to define your values and transmit those values to your staff. Shortcuts in quality and safety do not lead to good financial results nor to good outcomes. In the example of the ceiling leak in the OR described in Chapter Ten, preventive maintenance would have cost far less than closing several ORs for several days while the roof and ceilings were being repaired. Preventive maintenance might have eliminated risk to the patient's safety during surgery and avoided a costly and prolonged lawsuit—not to mention the adverse publicity apt to accompany an adverse event, which can harm the hospital's reputation.

Care depends on values. If your values and those of the organization you serve center on making money, you might well have felt pressured to open the OR prematurely. However, if you and your organization value patient safety, a full exploration of the causes of the leak would be first and foremost. In this example, a good manager would honestly explain to the patient and family what occurred, fill out an incident report, contact Engineering to locate the source of the problem and assess if other ORs were at risk, report to the safety officer, and contact the CEO. Honest and open communication, integrity, and accountability provide the best approach to handling a difficult situation. Good processes prevent unnecessary incidents, and knowing how to evaluate your service through the PDCA methodology helps you monitor the quality of care you deliver to every patient.

Good care is efficient and cost-effective care. We have tried to describe tools that you can use to assess the efficiency and effectiveness of your unit or service, and to help you develop the mindset to understand the continuum of care and the interrelatedness of services. Quality data can help you determine if you have an appropriate utilization of resources. If, for example, your patients cannot be discharged in a timely way because they have skin ulcers or their pneumonia is inadequately medicated, or their physical mobility is unexpectedly impaired due to a fall, LOS goes up, medication and other costly services increase, and no one is satisfied—not you, not your patients, not your hospital administration. Through analysis of variance data collected from clinical guidelines, managers can target which interventions were unmet, why they were unmet, and what effect that had on patient outcomes and on moving the patient efficiently through the hospital episode. Without information there can be no intelligent analysis or improvement.

A hospital is only as good as the services it delivers and the satisfaction of its patients. Good services and patient satisfaction depend on the manager accountable for their delivery. Monitoring care with the goal toward improvement has great value for managers, who can use them to illustrate that the provision of care is superior and also that it is cost-effective. Further, efficiency of care pleases the hospital administration because it is the right thing to do for the patients, and also because satisfying regulatory requirements and scoring well on surveys benefits the reputation and thus the success of the hospital.

Patients today are informed consumers of health care services. Since the future of health care involves the public reporting of quality indicators, it behooves managers to understand how to quantify, via data and measurements, the care they deliver so that outcomes are accurately reported. In addition, it can be useful to compare each unit's outcomes with others to define best practices. You can actually compare your services with other similar ones from across your region, or the nation, or even globally, to ascertain where you might have room to improve. Benchmarks give the manager perspective outside of the small world of the individual unit or even hospital.

Benchmarking, a concept that arose from the business sector as a way of determining how different branches of large organizations like IBM and Xerox performed, analyzes processes to define best practice. Once they establish best practice, these companies have a standard for comparison. In time, the idea of benchmarking and best practice was extended to include other comparable companies, so that, for example, billing practices could be compared not only internally, at different facilities within the same organization, but at many different types of businesses across the nation and around the world.

Comparison is useful because it helps an organization target goals. If one organization can accomplish great success, so can others. As the concept of benchmarking processes spread to health care, comparison data became available through state and national databases that monitor and collect quality indicators. Many health care organizations also have internal benchmarks, especially those hospitals that are part of larger health care systems, as is increasingly the case. If you track the rate of falls on your unit, or in your institution, or by service, and compare it to other units, institutions, or services, you can see if your rate is better or worse than the comparison rate. Ideally you know you want to have the lowest falls rate possible. The lower the rate, the better the care.

However, measurements, especially comparison measures, have to be used with caution, because defining a measure is such a complex process. It is imperative that you understand the measurement, the definition, the numerator and denominator, and the sample of a benchmark to ensure that you are comparing similar services or practices. Maybe the national benchmark is too general, or too limited, or based on averages rather than on best practice. Remember that to define a measure you want to compute events over opportunities. Statistics are easy to manipulate and many people have learned to use measures to make themselves look good. Managers who are invested in providing quality patient care use measurements carefully and with integrity. The objective is not to get a pat on the back but to serve your patient population.

Once you collect information via quality measurements, you need to analyze and interpret the information to determine whether improvements are indicated, and if already implemented, whether they are successful. Once again, care must be taken to ensure uniform data collection. If a unit or organization with which you are comparing your service has defined its indicator the same way you do, and defined its measurements the same way, and collected its data in the same way from a similar sample, a comparison is very useful. If you find an organization that seems to be doing something better than you are, according to the data, then you have a standard to reach toward. Benchmarks ensure that you don't become complacent.

If you think you have a good process in place in caring for patients, your measurements, over time, should confirm that the process is stable. Quality management tools such as control charts allow you to keep track of the stability of your processes. If you implement a new practice, the best way to assure yourself that it is successful is to measure the results carefully, again over time. If the data show that the problem you're trying to address decreases, your improvements may be responsible. If the rate stays high, you may have to introduce other processes, perhaps improved orientation or education. Improvements depend on the data.

If over time your careful measurements reveal a lack of improvement, you may want to use other quality tools to analyze your processes—

a fishbone diagram, flow chart, or FMEA can help you understand why the care isn't better and identify any weaknesses or risk points in the process. Once you identify the problems, use the PDCA methodology to develop and monitor the improvement processes. If you are pleased with your data, look around. Are you really the best? Don't you want to be? There is always room for improvement.

It is not always necessary to do a PDCA, however. If you know of a best practice that seems suitable for your service, try and adopt it. In our health care system, when one hospital implements a successful improvement, results are communicated through the committee structure. The Board expects that other hospitals will adopt the best practice and tailor it to their own needs. Identifying a best practice provides a valuable educational opportunity also. Ask your staff why that practice was best. Determine what is different from the way your unit provides that service. It is sometimes impractical or impossible to adopt a best practice because of financial or environmental factors. If that is the case, the challenge is to try and adapt that practice to your situation.

When your manager wants proof that you are doing a good job, or when an administrator wants to know how you are coping with your budgetary restrictions, providing data encompassing an awareness of benchmarks and best practices makes a great deal of sense. When a surveyor scrutinizes the care you deliver and compares it to care delivered throughout the nation, an awareness of benchmarks and best practice is impressive. Your work is always being evaluated somehow, by someone, including your patients. Having the right data will help you communicate effectively to your superiors and to your staff. Data can show that you know what you are doing and have set the bar high for your performance.

Our health system has been recognized through various professional publications and national conferences as having developed best practices in numerous procedures and services. The Quality Management Department receives calls from all over the world asking for help, advice, tools, and instruction, and we are pleased to share what we have learned. If you read or hear about a system or facility with patients similar to your own that is doing something better than you are, as confirmed through data, contact its management for information. In addition to the media, professional publications, and professional conferences, specialized societies and organizations often provide useful information. In fact you'll find a huge amount of information available. Best practices are not kept secret.

Throughout this book we have encouraged managers to recognize the value of communication in promoting quality care. Interestingly, just as poor communication is usually implicated in an error, good communication is integral to best practices. Working together and sharing information improves the process of care.

Communication, interaction, and sharing information increase when working within a quality management structure because quality pervades every department's function—which is to do the right thing well and provide patients with safe and excellent care. Quality management processes help managers monitor that care and serve as the glue to unite departments within the hospital and also hospitals that are part of larger health care systems. Individual cultures, whatever they may be, all have quality care in common.

A manager's job is dynamic, never static, moving always toward ongoing change and constant improvement. Our goal has been to make a case for change, and not simply a case but a course of action, exposing you to a plan or program where change can occur. To provide excellent service, new and creative ideas have to be presented on a welcome platform. You want to challenge your staff—and even yourself—to initiate improvements, rather than waiting for instructions from your manager or your administration. Your service and the patients you serve deserve your initiative. Today's health care environment supports change as hospitals are held accountable for the delivery of quality services, improved results, a safer environment, and meeting patient expectations regarding the services rendered.

This is a handbook for caregivers who want to acquire the tools they need to do the best job possible, and to understand the methods and theories that will enable them to do their jobs most successfully. Incorporating quality management methods into the daily working of your unit will help you identify what processes need change and allow you to sustain the change over time.

The health care business is about people providing services to other people who are in need of those services. If you have the knowledge and the tools to evaluate, measure, analyze, and improve your services, and you impart that knowledge to your staff, your unit will be more effective, and your patients will be better cared for. Administrative goals, patient expectations, regulatory requirements, and your own desire to deliver quality care will be well met.

Things to Think About

- Because of your use and understanding of quality methodologies, you have been promoted. Write a description of the skills and abilities you want to see in the manager chosen to replace you.

~~~ Bibliography

Agency for Health Care Policy and Research. *Clinical Practice Guidelines No. 3*. Rockville, Md.: U.S. Department of Health and Human Services, 1994.

Aguayo, R. *Dr. Deming: The American Who Taught the Japanese About Quality*. New York: Simon & Schuster, 1990.

Berwick, D. M. "Continuous Improvement as an Ideal in Health Care." In N. O. Graham (ed.), *Quality in Health Care: Theory, Application, and Evolution*. Gaithersburg, Md.: Aspen, 1995.

Dlugacz, Y. D., Restifo, A., Scanlon, K. A., Nelson, K., Fried, A. M., Hirsch, B., Delman, M., Zenn, R. D., Selzer, J., and Greenwood, A. "Safety Strategies to Prevent Suicide in Multiple Health Care Environments." *Joint Commission Journal on Quality and Safety*, 2003, *29*(6), 267–277.

Dlugacz, Y. D., Stier, L., and Greenwood, A. "Changing the System: A Quality Management Approach to Pressure Injuries." *Journal of Healthcare Quality*, 2001, *23*(5), 15–19.

Dlugacz, Y. D., Stier, L., Lustbader, D., Jacobs, M. C., Hussein, E., and Greenwood, A. "A Quality Approach to Critical Care." *Joint Commission Journal on Quality Improvement*, 2002, *28*(8), 419–434.

Donabedian, A. *Benefits in Medical Care Programs*. Cambridge, Mass.: Harvard University Press, 1976.

Donabedian, A. "The Role of Outcomes in Quality Assessment and Assurance." In N. O. Graham (ed.), *Quality in Health Care: Theory, Application, and Evolution*. Gaithersburg, Md.: Aspen, 1995.

Epstein, A. A. "The Outcomes Movement: Will It Get Us Where We Want to Go?" In N. O. Graham (ed.), *Quality in Health Care: Theory, Application, and Evolution*. Gaithersburg, Md.: Aspen, 1995.

Goonan, J. (ed.). *The Juran Prescription: Clinical Quality Management*. San Francisco: Jossey-Bass, 1995.

Graham, N. O. "Quality Trends in Health Care." In N. O. Graham (ed.), *Quality in Health Care: Theory, Application, and Evolution*. Gaithersburg, Md.: Aspen, 1995.

Hiam, A. *Closing the Quality Gap: Lessons from America's Leading Companies.* Upper Saddle River, N.J.: Prentice Hall, 1992.

Horn, S. D. (ed.). *Clinical Practice Improvement Methodology: Implementation and Evaluation,* Vol. 2. New York: Faulkner & Gray, 1997.

Ignatavicius, D. D., and Hausman, K. A. *Clinical Pathways for Collaborative Practice.* Philadelphia, Pa.: Saunders, 1995.

Institute of Medicine (ed.). *Crossing the Quality Chasm: A New Health System for the 21st Century.* Washington, D.C.: National Academy Press, 2001.

Joint Commission Resources. *National Library of Healthcare Indicators: Health Plan and Network Edition.* Oakbrook Terrace, Ill.: Joint Commission on Accreditation of Healthcare Organizations, 1997.

Joint Commission Resources. *Sentinel Event Alert, Issue Six.* Oakbrook Terrace, Ill.: Joint Commission on Accreditation of Healthcare Organizations, 1998.

Joint Commission Resources. *Florence Nightingale: Measuring Hospital Outcomes.* Oakbrook Terrace, Ill.: Joint Commission on Accreditation of Healthcare Organizations, 1999.

Joint Commission Resources. *Selecting and Implementing Clinical Practice Guidelines in Hospitals.* Oakbrook Terrace, Ill.: Joint Commission on Accreditation of Healthcare Organizations, 2000.

Joint Commission Resources. *Managing Performance Measurement Data in Health Care.* Oakbrook Terrace, Ill.: Joint Commission on Accreditation of Healthcare Organizations, 2001.

Joint Commission Resources. *Failure Mode and Effects Analysis in Health Care: Proactive Risk Reduction.* Oakbrook Terrace, Ill.: Joint Commission on Accreditation of Healthcare Organizations, 2002.

Joint Commission Resources. *From Practice to Paper: Documentation for Hospitals.* Oakbrook Terrace, Ill.: Joint Commission on Accreditation of Healthcare Organizations, 2002.

Joint Commission Resources. *Hospital Accreditation Standards.* Oakbrook Terrace, Ill.: Joint Commission on Accreditation of Healthcare Organizations, 2002.

Juran, J. M. *Juran on Quality by Design: The New Steps for Planning Quality into Goods and Services.* New York: Free Press, 1992.

Katz, J. M., and Green, E. *Managing Quality: A Guide to System-Wide Performance Management in Health Care.* St. Louis, Mo.: Mosby, 1997.

Kohn, L. T., Corrigan, J. M., and Donaldson, M. S. (eds.). *To Err Is Human: Building a Safer Health System.* Washington, D.C.: National Academy Press, 1999.

Landers, P. "Industry Urges Action on Health Costs." *Wall Street Journal,* June 11, 2002.

Margolis, C. Z. *Implementing Clinical Practice Guidelines.* Chicago: AHA Press, 1999.

Medical Quality Management Sourcebook 2000 Edition: A Comprehensive Guide to Standardizing Quality Measurement and Improving Care. New York: Faulkner & Gray, 1999.

Milstein, A., and others. "Improving the Safety of Health Care: The Leapfrog Initiative. The Leapfrog Group." *Effective Clinical Practice,* 2000, *5,* 313–316.

National Association for Healthcare Quality. *Guide to Quality Management.* (8th ed.) Glenview, Ill.: National Association for Healthcare Quality, 1998.

Parsons, T. *The Social System.* New York: Free Press, 1951.

Salkind, N. J. *Statistics for People Who (Think They) Hate Statistics.* Thousand Oaks, Calif.: Sage, 2000.

Senge, P. "Building Learning Organizations." In N. O. Graham (ed.), *Quality in Health Care: Theory, Application, and Evolution.* Gaithersburg, Md.: Aspen, 1995.

Shewhart, W. A. *Economic Control of Quality of Manufactured Product.* New York: Van Nostrand, 1931.

Spath, P. L. (ed.). *Beyond Clinical Paths: Advanced Tools for Outcomes Management.* Chicago: AHA Press, 1997.

Spath, P. L. "Reducing Errors Through Work System Improvements." In P. L. Spath (ed.), *Error Reduction in Health Care: A Systems Approach to Improving Patient Safety.* San Francisco: Jossey-Bass, 2000.

—•— Index